LEARNING HUM

A Guide for Nurses

We shall not cease from exploration
And the end of all our exploring
Will be to arrive where we started
And know the place for the first time.

T. S. Eliot

LEARNING HUMAN SKILLS

A Guide for Nurses

PHILIP BURNARD
MSc RMN RGN Dip N Cert Ed RNT

Lecturer in Nursing
Department of Nursing Studies
University of Wales College of Medicine

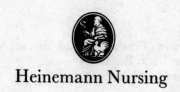

Heinemann Nursing

For Sally, Aaron and Rebecca

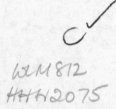
Heinemann Nursing
An imprint of Heinemann Professional Publishing Ltd
Halley Court, Jordan Hill, Oxford OX2 8EJ

OXFORD   LONDON   SINGAPORE
NAIROBI   IBADAN   KINGSTON

First published 1985
Reprinted 1986, 1988

© Philip Burnard 1985

ISBN 0 433 04905 7

Typeset by Eta Services (Typesetters) Ltd, Beccles, Suffolk
Printed and bound in Great Britain by
Biddles Ltd, Guildford and King's Lynn

CONTENTS

ACKNOWLEDGEMENTS

This book could not have been written without the help and experience of a considerable number of people. I am indebted to a great number of learner nurses, past and present, from whom I have learned about the practice of the experiential approach to nurse education. Thanks are also offered to Charles Bailey, Rita Strutt, Femi Ayoola and Jonathan Ooi, my colleagues at the School of Nursing, Netherne Hospital, Coulsdon, Surrey.

Particular thanks go to John Heron, Educational Consultant, British Postgraduate Medical Federation, University of London, for all his help and for his inspiration for much of the content of this book.

A problem arises out of the preparation of a book containing many experiential exercises. It is often difficult to trace the original source of such exercises. Often they are learned through participation in courses and workshops. I have tried to acknowledge sources wherever possible and gratefully thank the many people from whom I have learned experientially. A short list of these includes: Dolores Bate, Meg Bond, Gunna Dietrich, John Evans, John Heron, James Kilty, Malcolm Parlett and Dick Saxton. I am also particularly grateful to Dr Peter Jarvis, Dr Geoffrey Easting and Dr Alan Chadwick of the Department of Educational Studies, University of Surrey.

Every author depends upon a good relationship with their publisher. I am extremely grateful for the help and support that I have received from Ms Cathy Watson of William Heinemann Medical Books Ltd. Particular thanks go to Mrs Clare Horn, without whose skills and patience the typescript would not have been produced. I am also grateful to Ginny D'Santos for her work on the illustrations.

Finally, and most importantly, my gratitude goes to my wife, Sally and my children, Aaron and Rebecca, who have always been supportive, interested and helpful throughout the project.

As with all writing, any faults that exist in the theory or preparation of the book remain mine.

Philip Burnard

The extract from 'Little Gidding' is reprinted by permission of Faber & Faber Ltd, from *Four Quartets* by T. S. Eliot.

INTRODUCTION

This book has two aims. The first is to provide nurses with a clear and concise theoretical framework for understanding the concepts of self-awareness and experiential learning; the second is to offer a range of practical exercises for developing human skills: self-awareness, interpersonal and group skills. Self-awareness, as a vital prerequisite for the development of all other human skills, is a recurrent theme throughout the book.

It is hoped that the book will be of value to a wide range of nurses, from students in training to nurse tutors, nurse therapists and senior nurses. It is aimed at all spheres of nursing: general, psychiatric and mental handicap, as human skills are important in each. The book may also be an aid to curriculum developers and a source book for students on degree and higher education courses in nursing.

The book is fully referenced throughout so that the ideas presented can be developed further. Other books of particular relevance are recommended at the end of each chapter.

The book, then, is about self-exploration to a practical end, a process that is vital for anyone engaged in close involvement with other people. Nursing is essentially about interpersonal relationships. Every nursing situation, whether in the ward, in the home or in the school of nursing, requires the ability to relate skilfully to others. In order to develop such skill, the nurse needs to be self-aware. Unlike more technical skills, human or interpersonal skills demand a direct investment of self. In caring for others, in dealing with colleagues and in learning in the school of nursing, we are giving something directly of ourselves. Thus we must get to know ourselves better.

There are many ways in which nurses may develop such awareness. In the everyday nurse/patient encounter they may discover, if they listen, something about themselves. Patients and colleagues are constantly, if indirectly, offering feedback on our performance. In this sense we define ourselves through other people. People are telling us who we are. When a nurse is complimented on nursing practice or criticised for failure to complete a task, that process of self-definition is taking place.

In listening to what is said, and to what is implicit in what is being said, the nurse can gain new insights through which to modify or develop his or her behaviour. Self-awareness can also be developed through introspection, through examining inner thoughts and feelings. Such introspection need not be a morbid, indulgent process but a vital, inspirational act which may form the basis of decision making and skills development. A third pathway to self-awareness in interpersonal relationships is self-monitoring. By paying careful attention to what they are doing, how they are using and presenting themselves, nurses can learn the skill of enhancing their verbal and non-verbal behaviour.

Unfortunately, what often happens is that nurses notice what is happening around them—to patients, to colleagues or to the environment—but pay little attention to what happens to themselves. This attention only to others may be seen as true altruism, true concern for others, but by paying attention to themselves and becoming more skilled at self-management, nurses can enhance such altruism. Without self-awareness, the nurse is missing out half of any interaction with another person; with self-awareness that nurse is aware both of the other person and of him- or herself. Such awareness can be used to enhance the therapeutic relationship that exists between nurse and patient or the working and learning relationship that exists between the nurse and other professional colleagues.

This book offers an explanation of what self-awareness is and how it may be developed. It also offers a clear model of experiential learning: the process of learning through personal experience. Self-awareness is a personal issue; it cannot be taught through lectures, debates or other traditional teaching methods. Indeed, it cannot be *taught*, it can only be *learned*, using personal experience as the touchstone.

The book is in two halves. Part One offers a theoretical outline of the concepts of self-awareness and of experiential learning. In this section, the two issues are explored and explained in relation to the nursing profession. Part Two offers a variety of experiential exercises for developing self-awareness in interpersonal encounters. The exercises are related to counselling and group skills as well as to more general aspects of human relationships. The counselling skills exercises may be equated with day-to-day encounters between two people: the nurse in conversation with a patient, the tutor in discussion with a student. The group section may be taken to parallel any meeting between more than two people: the nursing report, ward meetings, tutorials and discussion groups in the school of nursing. This is not to say that counselling *is the same as* any meeting of two people, nor to argue that any collection of people may be called a 'group', but to note that there are vital similarities between all types of human relationships. These similarities are the essence of encounters with others; they constitute what it is to be human and to be sociable beings. The labels 'counselling' and 'groups' should not be too distracting. At best they serve as a guide to understanding aspects of relationships. Once the skills within the two categories have been learnt, they can be more widely applied and the labels can be discarded.

The exercises in Part Two are clearly laid out so that they can be used by a wide variety of nurses. The nurse who wishes to develop self-awareness and interpersonal skills in his or her own time will find exercises that can be carried out by one person. However, feedback from others is a vital aid to the learning process in this field, and many of the exercises are therefore designed to be carried out in groups. Student nurses may wish to use them in peer groups and nurse tutors will find many of the exercises useful in planning interpersonal skills workshops. Guidelines are offered for the use of the exercises and for group facilitation.

The exercises in the book can only be a beginning. Once they have been used and reused in a variety of settings, it is the responsibility of the individual nurse to carry over what has been learned into the practical nursing situation. In this respect self-awareness cannot be seen as a product. No nurse can claim to have achieved self-awareness. It is a continuous and sometimes faltering process. Learning through experience is a dynamic, ever-changing process that can be enhanced by the use of exercises, but such exercises are not an end in themselves. As self-awareness develops, however, the exercises may be adapted and modified to explore further issues. The innovative nurse tutor may find ways of using the exercises to explore particular nursing situations that are specific to particular wards and departments. Student nurses may wish to modify certain exercises in order to make personal discoveries or to develop interpersonal skills gained so far. Often, however, the best exercises are those that individuals and groups make up for themselves; that amplify and illustrate particular personal and group issues that are specific to them. The exercises in this book should be practical in that they bring about new development and change.

Finally, it is hoped that the exercises will prove to be enjoyable. Self-discovery can be lighthearted as well as hard work! Typically, the exercises will work best when they are carried out in an environment which is supportive but not too earnest. Human relationships are, after all, enjoyable, or nursing would not be the satisfying occupation that it is.

The book is, then, an introduction to the concepts of self-awareness, interpersonal skills and experiential learning; it can be used as a training manual for nurse tutors and trainers in post-basic and in-service nurse education; it can be taken into the classroom as a guide for conducting exercises; and it can be used by students as part of a programme of self-exploration and self-development.

PART ONE

CHAPTER ONE

The Self and Self-awareness

The self

The concept of self is complex. What do we mean when we talk of the self? To what are we referring when we use expressions such as—'speaking for myself...'? Can we talk of a 'real' self as opposed to something we adopt as a mask, as a front, with which to face the world: a 'false' self? Is it possible to devise a concrete, practical map of the self?

Questions like these have interested philosophers, psychologists and theologians for centuries. The existential school of philosophy discusses the issue of the self under the heading of 'ontology': the study of being. The self in this context is something more than just physical, bodily existence. It is the fact of being a conscious, knowing human being. Sartre (1956) talks of authenticity—the state of true and honest presentation of being. The authentic person, for Sartre, consistently acts in accordance with their own values, wishes and feelings, making no attempt to play-act or to adopt a façade, but acting as honestly and genuinely as possible. R. D. Laing (1959) took this notion further when he offered the idea of a 'true' and 'false' self. The true self is the inner, private sense of self. The false self is the outer, often pretending sense of self. According to Laing, the true self often watches what the false self is doing and a sense of contempt is experienced. The false self is often compliant to the needs of others and can be artificial and insincere. In Sartre's terms, the false self acts inauthentically. The person who has a strong sense of the 'real' self, who is able to act authentically and honestly, is deemed by Laing to have ontological security: security of being. Such security can enable the individual to make decisions, to feel able to act rather than feeling acted upon, and generally to feel more autonomous.

We can see examples of Sartre's and Laing's ideas in practice within the context of nursing. If we notice that we are 'acting the role of nurse' in talking with patients, rather than being ourselves, then we are behaving in an inauthentic manner. This is not a plea for an unprofessional manner, but to note that there is a world of difference between the nurse who is genuine, open and sincere, yet still professional, and the nurse who adopts a professional façade, an artificial manner, and who fools no one—neither themselves, their colleagues nor their patients. The nurse who becomes self-aware can monitor their behaviour and note any tendency towards adopting such a veneer.

Psychologists have approached the concept of self from a variety of points of view. Some have attempted to analyse out the factors that go to make up the self rather in the way that a cook might try to discover the ingredients that have gone into a cake. Others have argued that there are certain consistent aspects of the self that determine to some extent the way in which we conduct and live our lives. Psychoanalytical theory, for instance, argues that early childhood experiences profoundly affect and shape the self, determining how as adults we react to the world about us. Childhood experiences lay foundations of the self which may be modified by experience but which nevertheless stay constant throughout life. Such a view is 'deterministic': our present sense of self is determined by earlier life experiences; and we are shaped to a greater or lesser degree by our childhoods.

Other psychological theorists acknowledge problems with reductionist theories—theories that attempt to analyse the self into parts or individual aspects. They prefer to view the self from a holistic or gestalt perspective. The gestalt approach argues that the whole or totality of the self is always something different from, or larger than, the sum of the aspects that make it up. Just as we cannot discover the true nature of a piece of music by examining the piece note by note, neither can we understand the self by analysing it into separate aspects.

So we have a problem; if it is the case that the self-as-a-whole is necessarily more than the sum of its individual parts, how do we study the self without losing sight of the whole? The answer is that we must proceed with caution. In examining one small aspect of self, we must always bear in mind the larger context. Similarly, any change to one aspect of self will have a domino or knock-on effect with other aspects and thus the whole.

It is worth noting at this point that we do not exist in isolation. What we are and who we are depends, to a very large extent, upon the other people with whom we live, work and relate. Our sense of self depends upon the reports about us that we receive from others. As nurses, we rely on patients, colleagues and tutors offering us both positive and negative feedback on our performance. Such feedback is slowly absorbed by the individual, modifying and enhancing the sense of self. Thus it seems sensible to consider the idea of self-exploration and self-awareness training in the company of others. Whilst some of the exercises in the second section of this book can be carried out in isolation, many are group activities. Such exercises allow both personal experience and reports from others. The combination of individual and group experience is a vital one if the self-awareness developed is to be accurate and realistic.

Taking into account this self-in-relation-to-others concept, some writers have postulated a transpersonal dimension to the self. The word transpersonal refers to that which unites all persons. Jung (1978), for example, argued for the existence of the 'collective unconscious', a domain that contains all human experience, both past and present, to which we all have access. Supporting arguments for the existence of this collective unconscious include the fact of synchronicity or meaningful coincidence. We may be thinking of someone and they telephone us, or we are about to say something and the person we are with says exactly the same thing. These are examples of synchronous events. The appearance of symbols in dreams is also offered as evidence for the collective unconscious: Jung maintained that certain types of symbols, circles and crosses, for example, occur through the ages in all parts of the world and in many contexts. He felt that this could not be dismissed. Further, these symbols often appear in our dreams and Jung argued that such appearances were made possible through our tapping the collective unconscious.

Other writers have considered that meditation and altered states of consciousness can aid our appreciation of the transpersonal domain (see for example Heron, 1975a; Masters and Houston, 1973). Heron (1981a) has also suggested a new research method for the exploration of the transpersonal domain. This more spiritual area of the person may be a fruitful one to explore. What is important, however, is that the nurse who wishes to do this is first clear of his or her own spiritual beliefs and values. The first step towards examining the transpersonal dimension of the self may be just this: the clarification and examination of theological and religious beliefs. Such clarification can enhance self-awareness and can in the process help the nurse to help others to clarify their religious ideas. The transpersonal and spiritual aspect of the person remains largely unexplored in both the nursing literature and nursing practice. It is only as individual nurses examine their own thoughts and feelings on the matter that the profession as a whole can move towards change in this area.

Here, too, lies the more significant value of self-awareness training. Such training can never be just for the individual's own development and personal satisfaction. At its best, self-awareness leads us to greater understanding of other people. Rather than becoming selfish and self-centred, we can use self-understanding to aid the therapeutic process in others, whether in the field of general, mental handicap or psychiatric nursing.

What, then, is a concept of self that is concrete, practical and readily available for use? In its simplest form, the self can be seen as made up of three areas or focuses of interest. Figure 1.1 shows these three domains: thoughts, feelings and behaviour. By thoughts is meant the process of ideas, puzzlement, problem-solving that makes up our mental life. By feelings is meant the emotional aspects of our being: happiness, grief, love, anger, etc. Behaviour refers to any action that we carry out and also to the spoken word and to what is usually referred to as non-verbal be-

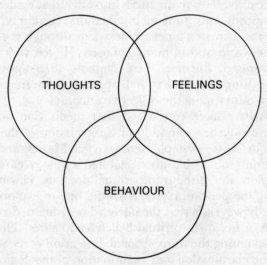

Fig. 1.1 *Simple model of the self.*

haviour: eye contact, facial expression, gestures, proximity to others, etc. (These non-verbal aspects will be examined more closely in another section.) All three aspects of the self, in this simple model, overlap. We cannot think without in some way feeling and behaving. As we think, we become aware of pleasant or irritating feelings and this leads to often very small but nevertheless notice-able changes in our behaviour. If someone is in the room with you now, just notice them and observe how you can tell that they are thinking. You will observe changes in eye contact, or facial expression, or, perhaps, arm and leg movements. Their expression will also indicate something of their mood and thus access is made to the domain of feeling.

This interrelatedness of the domains of thoughts, feelings and behaviour is noticeable from any other starting point. If we pon-der for a moment on how we are feeling, such pondering involves thinking and, in turn, a change in our behaviour. Here then is a starting point for approaching the study of the self. We may study each of the domains and come to know something more about ourselves. As we study each domain and appreciate the connec-tion between all three we gradually peel back the layers to a deeper understanding of the self. The exercises in the second half of this book will focus on all three domains, although certain exer-cises will concentrate more on one than on the others. Once again, the point is clear: all aspects of self are related to each other. To make a change in one aspect is to affect all the others.

This then is a simple model of the self. Figure 1.2 offers a more complex model which, whilst compatible with the first, opens up the domains and expands them. If the first model was a basic work-ing model, this is a development of that model. It allows for more thinking and experiencing of a greater variety of aspects of the self. It incorporates Jung's work on the four aspects of human ex-perience: thinking, feeling, sensing and intuiting (Jung, 1978) and also an adaptation of Laing's (1959) concept of the real and false self. This concept describes the inner and outer aspects of the self.

This model is divided into two parts. The outer, public aspect of the self is what others see of us. The inner, private aspect is what goes on in our heads and bodies. In one sense, the outer experi-ence is what other people are most familiar with. We communi-cate the inner experience through the outer. Our thoughts and feelings are all communicated through this outer experience of be-haviour. Of what does it consist?

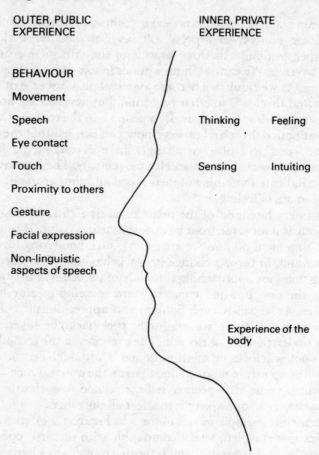

OUTER, PUBLIC
EXPERIENCE

INNER, PRIVATE
EXPERIENCE

BEHAVIOUR

Movement

Speech   Thinking   Feeling

Eye contact

Touch   Sensing   Intuiting

Proximity to others

Gesture

Facial expression

Non-linguistic
aspects of speech

Experience of the
body

Fig. 1.2   *A comprehensive model of the self.*

The outer experience

At the most obvious level, behaviour consists of body movements:
the turn of the head, the crossing of arms and legs, walking and
running, and so on. At a more subtle level, however, the issue
becomes more involved. We may note a whole variety of more
subtle behaviours that convey the inner sense of self. First then, is
the behaviour we call speech. Clearly what we say, the words and
phrases we use, are a potent means by which we convey thoughts
and feelings to others. How we come to choose *these* particular

words and phrases, however, depends upon our past experiences, our education, our social position, our attitudes, values and beliefs, and the company that we are in when we use those words. Running alongside speech are the non-linguistic aspects of speech: timing, pacing, volume, 'mm's', the use of silence, and so on. The use of such non-linguistic aspects of communication can be potent in conveying our inner selves to others.

When we talk to others we invariably look at them. As Heron (1970) notes there can be a wide variety in the intensity, amount and quality of eye contact. When we are embarrassed or upset, for instance, we make less eye contact. When we are emotionally close to another person, our eye contact is often sustained. We can learn to become conscious of our use of what must be the most powerful aspect of communication and to monitor the amount and quality of our eye contact.

Touch in relation to others is another aspect of our outer experience. Typically we touch more those people to whom we are close: members of the family, lovers and very close friends. Certainly, nursing involves a high degree of this personal aspect of human interaction and it is important that, as with eye contact, nurses learn to monitor and consciously choose the amount of touch they use.

When we relate to others, the fact of communicating means that we must necessarily be near them. How near we sit or stand in relation to others is determined by a number of factors—the level of intimacy we have with them, our relationship with them and whether or not we are dominant or submissive in that relationship (Brown, 1965). In the nursing profession, nurses tend to be in a dominant role *vis à vis* their patients, and will tend, therefore, to stand closer to their patients than would be the case in ordinary day-to-day relationships. Desmond Morris (1978) suggests the useful idea that we are surrounded by an invisible circle or bubble which may only be crossed by certain other individuals. If people accidentally break through the circle and touch us, we tend to withdraw quickly often to the embarrassment of both parties. The issue of proximity to others needs careful consideration. We need to become aware of how close or distant we like to be in relation to others. We need to note also other people's preferences in this respect and to be sensitive to them. Once again, as we become more self-aware, so we gain more insight into the needs and wants of others.

One of the clearest indicators of our inner experience is our facial expression. Frowns and smiles can do much to convey the feelings that are being experienced inside. It is important, however, that facial expression and speech are congruent or matched. We have all experienced the person who *says* that they are cheerful or upset but whose facial expression says otherwise. Bandler and Grinder (1975) note that for the purposes of clear communication three aspects of our outer behaviour must match: general body position, content of speech, and facial expression. If one or more of these three are mismatched, then our communication will be received by others as confusing. Thus if we *say* to others that we are cheerful but shrug our shoulders and have an unhappy expression on our face, the message will be unclear. Much useful work can be done on this aspect of our outer experience. We can learn to be congruent in our communication with others and to ensure that our speech, behaviour and facial expression all clearly indicate the same thing. In our nursing experience this must surely be one of the major aspects of nurse/patient interaction. Can we be sure that we are conveying to our patient the message that we intend? When we use reassuring phrases are we also being reassuring in our gestures and expression? This concept of congruence is one example of how the notion of self-awareness can increase our effectiveness in dealing with others. It is insufficient just to *say* what we mean. We must be *seen* to express it as well.

Two issues become clear from this analysis of the outer aspect of self. We can become aware of our use of speech, eye contact, touch, proximity to others, gesture, facial expression and non-linguistic aspects of speech, as a means of deepening our understanding of ourselves. On the other hand, by becoming conscious of how we use those verbal and non-verbal behaviours, we can more skilfully use them to enhance our contact with others. We can increase our interpersonal skills by intentionally using ourselves as an instrument. Heron uses the expression 'conscious use of the self' (Heron, 1973) to convey this concept. This is not to say that such use of the self should take place in a mechanical, artificial manner. To act in this way would be to act inauthentically. It is vital that this use of overt, noticeable behaviour is applied after inner reflection on values, beliefs and attitudes. To act without care and thought for others would be less than human. To act *consciously* with due feeling for others enhances the quality of care that is offered to patients in every nursing situation.

The inner experience

The inner, private experience in this model may be divided into aspects of mental functioning—thinking, feeling, sensing and intuiting—and the experience of the body. Clearly, the division of these aspects into two groups in this way is artificial, as both mental and physical events are interrelated. As Searle (1983) points out, a mental event is also a physical event. To think that it is not is to perpetuate the old philosophical problem of mind/body dualism. This is sometimes known as Cartesian dualism after the philosopher René Descartes, who believed that mental and physical events were to be considered differently. Today, the tendency is towards healing this split and interest is growing in the concepts of holistic nursing and holistic medicine—both of which treat mind and body together. Certainly, any concept of the self must take into account the mind and the body as a totality.

The thinking dimension

In the present model, thinking refers to all the aspects, logical and illogical, of our mental processes. One moment's reflection on thinking will reveal that it is not a linear process. We do not think in sentences or even in a series of phrases. The process is much more haphazard than that. The technique of 'free-association' used in psychoanalysis demonstrates the apparently random nature of some of our thinking. Free association demands that the individual verbalises whatever comes into their mind, without any attempt at censoring. Try to attempt to do this: the process is difficult certainly and often impossible. The reasons for this difficulty are outlined in the psychoanalytic literature and such theory can offer insights into the genesis and nature of thought processes. Clearly not everyone wants or can afford psychoanalysis but its ideas can be useful in attempting to understand thinking.

Interestingly, the domain of thinking is more dominant in certain individuals. Certainly, thinking is highly rated in our culture and the educational system often concerns itself *only* with this mode. The domains of feeling, sensing and intuiting are invariably less well catered for. In nursing, however, we are concerned with feelings of all sorts, from pain to anxiety, from depression to elation. Understanding these feelings requires the use of dimensions other than thinking.

The feeling dimension

Feeling in this model refers to the emotional aspect of the person: love, joy, sadness, happiness, etc. Heron (1977a) notes four predominant aspects of emotion that are frequently denied in our society: anger, grief, fear and embarrassment. He argues that anger can be expressed through loud sound and shouting, grief through tears, fear through trembling, and embarrassment through laughter. The expression of pent-up emotion is called catharsis. Heron argues that we live in a non-cathartic society and the general tendency is to encourage people to control rather than express profound emotion. As a result, we carry around with us considerable unexpressed feeling that affects our self concept and our daily lives. If, on the other hand, we can learn to express that emotion, and methods for learning these skills will be discussed later, then we can become more open to experience, less anxious, and can exercise greater autonomy and freedom. Part of becoming self-aware entails discovery and exploring the emotional dimension—the often ignored domain.

Nurses are frequently called upon to deal with other people's emotion and there is a positive correlation between the way in which we can handle our own emotions and the way in which we can handle others' emotions. If we understand and can appropriately and freely express our own anger, grief, fear and embarrassment, we will be better able to handle those emotions in other people. Certainly other people's emotions affect us and stir up our own unexpressed feelings. A simple experiment will demonstrate this. Next time a programme on television moves you near to tears, turn off the set and allow yourself to cry. As you do so, reflect upon what you are crying about. It is highly likely that the issue causing the tears is a personal issue, not directly related to the television programme. Most people carry around with them this unexpressed emotion that lies just beneath the surface. Nurses who work in particularly emotional environments—children's wards, intensive care units and psychiatric units, for example—may wish to consider self-help methods of exploring their own catharsis. Co-counselling is one such method and a variety of others are discussed by Bond and Kilty (1982).

The sensing dimension

The sensing dimension of the model refers to inputs through the five special senses: touch, taste, smell, hearing, sight, and also to proprioceptive and kinaesthetic sense. Proprioception refers to our ability to know the position of our bodies and thus to know where we are in space. We do not, for instance, need to *think* about our body position for much of the time—we are fed that information by bundles of nerve fibres known as proprioceptors. Kinaesthetic sense refers to our sense of body movement. Again, this is a sense about which we do not normally have consciously to think. Clearly, however, we can make ourselves aware of any of the stated senses. Another simple experiment will demonstrate this. Stop reading for a moment and pay attention to everything that you can hear. Take in all the sounds around you: the more subtle as well as obvious. In doing so, you will notice how much of one particular sense is normally passed over, as unimportant and thus unnoticed. At times it is vital that our senses are selective and that extraneous sounds, images, smells and so on are filtered out of our consciousness but on the other hand, there are times when a more acute awareness of the senses can enhance our relationship with the world around us and with the people in that world. In developing our sense of sight, for example, we can begin to notice subtle changes in other people's expressions, body postures, eye contact and other aspects of non-verbal communication. Without that awareness we may miss a considerable amount of vital interpersonal information. In nursing the value of such awareness is clear. Nurses are trained to be observant in order to draw up clear care plans and to evaluate those plans. What is often not made so clear is *how* such observational skills are to be developed. Regular attention to the senses can enhance observational skills. Like any other skills training, the development of sensory awareness takes time and practice. Fortunately such training can be carried out by the individual on their own by just setting aside a part of each day to *notice* what is going on around them. Eventually such awareness, or 'staying awake' as it may be called, becomes part of the person. Through regular use of all their senses, that person becomes someone with more highly developed senses. The practical value of such training is clear: such a person is more observant, more accurate and more sensitive to subtle changes in other people and in the environment.

The intuitive dimension

The intuitive dimension is perhaps the most undervalued. Intuition refers to knowledge and insight that arrive independently of inputs from the senses. Ornstein (1975) who has studied the literature and research on the differences between the two sides of the brain, identifies intuition with the right side. He sees the two sides as having qualitatively different functions. The left side is concerned with cognitive (thought) processes and with rationality and logic. The right side is more to do with holism, creativity and intuition. If Ornstein is right, the implication is that if the intuitive aspect is developed further then both sides of the brain will be used optimally. Ornstein's argument is that the present Western culture is dominated by the left brain approach to education and development. He places intuition beyond mere intellectual understanding in terms of importance, and advocates the use of metaphors, allegories and Sufi fables as the means by which intuition can be developed.

Perhaps the intuitive aspect of the person is neglected through fear that it may not be trusted. It seems probable that everyone experiences intuitive thoughts and feelings, but that many fail to act on them or be guided by them. On the other hand, many aspects of nursing require a certain intuitive quality. In order to empathise with others, an ability intuitively to grasp what it is to experience what the other is feeling is vital. Certainly group work and counselling in psychiatric nursing depend upon it. Carl Rogers, the founder of client-centred counselling, notes that whenever he felt a 'hunch' about something that was happening in a counselling session, it invariably helped if he verbalised it (Rogers, 1967). Using intuition consciously and openly takes courage but used hand in hand with more traditional forms of thinking, it can enhance the nurse/patient relationship in a way that cold logic never can.

The experience of the body

The third aspect of the model of self-awareness is the experience of the body. If mind and body are directly interrelated, in fact inseparable, then any mental activity will affect the body and vice versa. It is notable, however, that much of the literature in nursing and medicine divides the person up into separate psychological and physiological entities. Indeed the two spheres are treated, typically, by different practitioners: general nurses care for physical ailments and psychiatric nurses for psychological problems. One moment's reflection, however, will reveal how artificial such a distinction is. The mind/body is a unified entity. Indeed we do not *have* a mind/body, we *are* our mind/body. Everything that we refer to as being part of our mind and body is part of our selves, even if it seems easier to refer to them at times as if they were merely attachments. Expressions such as 'I'm not happy with my body . . .', or 'I've got that sort of mind . . .', indicate how easy it is to talk about aspects of the self as though they were objects attached to the person.

Coming to notice body feelings takes time and patience. Of course, appreciation of inner bodily experiences is limited to some degree by the supply of sensory nerve endings to certain aspects of the body. Some parts are better served than others. On the other hand, it is easy to lose touch with those bodily sensations of which we may become aware. Before you read further, just take a moment to notice what is going on inside your body. What do you notice? Are there areas of muscular tension perhaps in the shoulders or the chest? Are the muscles of your stomach fully relaxed or do you pull your stomach in tightly? Can you become aware of feeling in your arms and legs? How is your breathing? Are you breathing deeply into your stomach or is your breathing light and shallow? What happens when you make changes to your body, when you relax sets of muscles or change your breathing?

All the information that can be gleaned from the body can enable us to appreciate something about our psychological status. Tension in sets of muscles, for instance, may be the first we know of the fact that we are generally tense or worried about something. Learning to 'listen' to the body can help us more accurately to assess our true feelings about ourselves and others. Wilhelm Reich (1949), a psychoanalyst who was particularly interested in the mind/body relationship, advanced the notion of 'character armour'. Reich maintained that our emotional feelings could get trapped within sets of muscles and consequently affected posture and movement. He maintained that direct manipulation of those sets of muscles could release the emotion trapped within them with characteristic catharsis. Such work on the body has become known as Reichian bodywork and can be a powerful and effective means of developing self-awareness through direct body contact. Similar but different methods of this sort, which involve direct physical contact include Rolfing (Rolf, 1973), bioenergetics (Lowen, 1967) and Feldenkrais (Feldenkrais, 1972), three bodywork methods that have developed out of Reich's original formulation. Less dramatic, but nevertheless valid methods of body/mind exploration and awareness include: massage, yoga, the martial arts, certain types of meditation, the Alexander technique (Alexander, 1969), dance and certain types of sport and exercise. Examples of meditative exercises are included in the second half of this book.

All these methods can enhance awareness of self through attention to changes in the body and thus create insight into psychological stages. They can also aid the development of awareness of body image. Observations of people in everyday life will reveal how frequently people walk around with lop-sided shoulders, a stooping gait, or even with either side of the face showing different expressions! These bodywork methods can enable the individual to develop more physical symmetry, a better posture, improved breathing and a healthier physical status generally. The advantages of these changes are clear and of particular value for the nurse. All aspects of nursing call for psychological and physical stamina and are taxing on the mind/body. These methods in combination with more traditional approaches to self-awareness can lead to a powerful and healthy approach to self care. Perhaps burnout, so frequently a problem of occupations that depend upon a high degree of human contact, can be prevented effectively through this mix of attention to the body and the mind.

What has been offered here is an integrated model of the self: a model that takes into account the outer, behavioural sense and the inner, mind/body sense of self. None of the three aspects is presented as more or less important than the others. In a sense too, the model must have its limitations. There are numerous and probably indefinable aspects of each person that cannot be accounted for in this way. It is vital, too, to remember that we are always selves-in-relation to others. How others see us, how we *think* they see us and how we act in relation to them are also, of themselves, aspects of the self. In being viewed by others and in our dealings with them, we are constantly redefining our own self concepts. The self is dynamic, flexible and changing. The model presented here offers some of the aspects of it that may fruitfully be explored as we attempt to improve our human skills—our skills in relating to each other as subject to subject.

Self-awareness

So far we have discussed what may be understood as a concept of self. A model has been outlined that takes account of the inner and outer aspects of the concept and which has attempted to marry the mind and the body. The question now arises: what are we to understand by the concept of self-awareness?

A first point that needs to be made here is that what is *not* being discussed is 'self-consciousness' in the everyday sense. To be self-conscious is to be embarrassed by our self-presentation, to be painfully aware of ourselves as observed by others. Sartre (1956) describes this well when he says that under the scrutinising gaze of another person, we are turned into an object, a 'thing'. It is our response to being treated in this way that causes us to become self-conscious. We realise that we are to a greater or lesser extent under the microscope. We are being examined by others in a way that makes us feel less than human. Clearly, for the very self-conscious person, this sense of being treated as an object is exaggerated by that person themselves. In being too acutely aware of other people's attention, they imagine themselves to be more acutely scrutinised than is actually the case. This is true, for instance of the adolescent, who imagines (probably falsely) that they are being looked at with highly critical eyes. Their own sense of insecurity is projected onto the world and they imagine that others view them as harshly and as critically as they view themselves.

Clearly, such self-consciousness is more of a hindrance than a help when it comes to relating to others, as any acutely shy person knows. Yet such self-consciousness is far removed from self-awareness, as we saw above, it often indicates a false or exaggerated self-concept.

Self-awareness refers to the gradual and continuous process of noticing and exploring aspects of the self, whether behavioural, psychological or physical, with the intention of developing personal and interpersonal understanding. Such awareness cannot be developed for its own sake; it is intimately bound up with our relationships with others. To become more aware of, and to have a deeper understanding of ourselves is to have a sharper and clearer picture of what is happening to others. In a sense, it is a process of discrimination. The more we can discriminate ourselves from others, the more we can understand our similarities. This curious paradox is the key to the importance of self-awareness training in the caring professions. If we are unaware and blind to our own selves, then we will remain blind to others. A rather crude illustration may serve to drive home this point. If I buy a red sweater, I immediately notice how many other people are wearing red sweaters—a fact of which I was not aware before the purchase. In noticing that fact about the others, I also notice other things about them. And so, if I let it, the process escalates. I can notice the more subtle differences between persons, but also their similarities. The point is that the process begins with me. I must first examine myself.

Such a process of examination requires patience and honesty. It is easy to fall into the trap of *interpreting* thoughts, feelings and behaviour, rather than (initially at least) merely noticing them. That interpretation comes logically *after* we have gathered the data, after we have clearly described to ourselves our present status. This stage in self-awareness training may be likened to the assessment phase of the nursing process. Information about the self is gathered in order to develop a clearer picture, before any attempt is made to problem solve, decide upon changes, or identify reasons for the way we are.

This approach may be described as phenomenological. Phenomenology is a branch of philosophy that is concerned with attempting to *describe* things as they appear to be without recourse to value-judgements about them. Thus, in the human context, a phenomenological approach to self-awareness training would concern itself purely with *describing* aspects of the self as they surface and become known. Such an approach demands that we suspend judgement on ourselves. Instead of acknowledging that a certain aspect of ourselves is good or bad, we merely note that it is so. The question of *why* it is the case or whether or not it *ought* to be the case can be dealt with at a later date when a more complete picture has emerged. Once we have more data at our disposal, the answers to such questions may become self-evident. To jump to hasty conclusions may be either (a) to be harshly over-critical of ourselves, or (b) to wreck the project altogether because we are disenchanted. Certainly, the road to self-awareness is not an easy one to tread, but the phenomenological approach can make it bearable.

This method, of description rather than interpretation, is of great value in group settings. When experiential learning is discussed in the next chapter, the notion of the phenomenological role of the facilitator will be discussed. In this role the facilitator of the group does not attempt to offer interpretations of what is happening in the group but limits him- or herself to description of events and encourages the group members to do the same. Indeed, such an approach may be carried through to nurse/patient interactions. To interpret what we imagine is the case for our patient is a precarious way to proceed. To describe what we observe of them, to them, is of greater value. As self-awareness develops, the need and temptation to *interpret* another person's behaviour may become less important. The problem with such analysis must always be that it will be coloured by our own experiences, feelings and thoughts. When we interpret other people's behaviour, we are invariably saying a great deal about ourselves. It is surely more valuable to understand ourselves first and avoid the temptation to offer dubious analyses of others.

Developing self-awareness

There are various routes towards self-awareness. Some invove introspection and some entail involvement with and feedback from other people. Any course leading towards self-awareness must contain both facets: the inner search and the observations of others. Clearly, introspection by itself can lead to a one-sided, totally subjective view of the self. It is difficult (though arguably not impossible) for the person working on their own to transcend themselves, to stand outside themselves and look back from an objective point of view. The introspective path is a totally subjective path. In order to balance that subjectivity, we need the view of others.

Before examining some of the methods of introspection and group work, it is useful to note one simple method of enhancing self-awareness: the process of noticing what we are doing, the process of self-monitoring. All that is involved here is staying conscious of what you are doing and what is happening to you. In other words, you 'stay awake' and develop the skill of keeping your attention focussed on your actions, both verbal and non-verbal. Such a process, whilst in theory simple, can in practice be quite difficult. It is easy to become distracted by inner thoughts and preoccupations so that our actions become automatic and unnoticed—even robotic. At this point it is useful to examine three zones of attention on which we can focus. Figure 1.3 shows these three zones. Zone 1 is the zone of having our attention focussed 'out'—on to our behaviour or on to the world outside ourselves. This is the zone that is being referred to above. To 'stay awake' in this context is to have our attention focussed outwards.

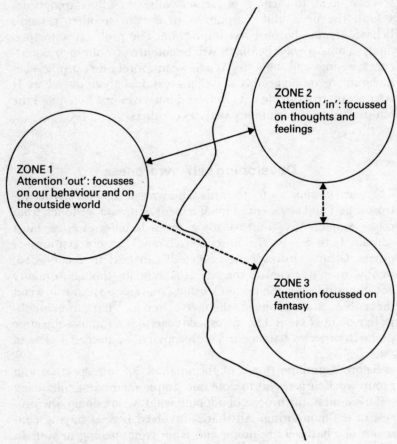

ZONE 2
Attention 'in': focussed on thoughts and feelings

ZONE 1
Attention 'out': focusses on our behaviour and on the outside world

ZONE 3
Attention focussed on fantasy

Fig. 1.3   *Possible zones of attention.*

There are some simple devices, borrowed from meditational practice, that can encourage, enhance or develop our ability to keep
our attention in that zone. Here is a particularly straightforward
one. Stop reading for a moment and allow your eyes to focus on an
object in the room that you are in: it may be a piece of furniture, a
picture or anything else that is to hand. Focus your attention on
that object and notice every detail of it: its contours, its colour, its
shape and so forth. Continue to do this for between thirty seconds
and one minute. Then discontinue your close observation. Notice
how your attention has shifted from thoughts and feelings on the
'inside', to what is going on outside yourself. The practice of this
simple exercise can help in getting and keeping attention 'out'.
With such focus of attention, it is easier to maintain a process of
self-monitoring. Further, it can be a very positive aid in helping us
to become more aware of others; if we are focussing our attention
outside ourselves, we are in a better position to notice what others
are saying and doing. From such a position we can really listen to
and take note of others.

Zones 2 and 3 in Figure 1.3 are the zones of introspection.
Inward focussing of attention (or 'attention in') can be useful as a
means of exploring thoughts, feelings and bodily sensations. Access to Zone 2 is very straightforward. Stop reading and close your
eyes. Allow your attention to range freely over what is going on in
your mind. Notice the things that you are thinking; notice how
you are feeling and then pay attention to any body sensations that
you have. What parts of your body are you aware of? What parts
can you not sense at all? Is there anything you can do in order to
become aware of those parts of the body? After one or two
minutes, open your eyes and switch your focus back to the outside
world. Notice whether such a switch is easy or difficult. The ability to shuttle between Zones 1 and 2 can be developed through
practice.

Zone 3 in the diagram involves fantasy. Fantasy refers to all our
thoughts and feelings that involve imagining or day-dreaming.
Notice how we so often have fantasies about both ourselves and
others that are in no way related to fact. We *imagine*, for instance,
what other people think of us; we *imagine* what sort of people other
people are. Often these imaginings or fantasies are based on very
flimsy evidence. On many occasions they are pure fantasy—they
have no grounding in fact at all! Differentiating between Zones 2
and 3 is particularly fruitful. If we acknowledge when we are

moving from the zone of logical, clear thinking (Zone 2) to the zone of fantasy (Zone 3), we develop a clearer picture of what goes on inside our heads and indeed, the nature of our thinking processes. This is not to denigrate the zone of fantasy, for it can help us to develop creativity and inspiration. It is vital, however, that we clearly separate fact from fantasy: clear thinking based on sound evidence from imagination and reverie.

Awareness of focus of attention and its shift between the three zones has implications for all aspects of nursing situations. The nurse who is able to keep attention directed out for long periods is likely to be more observant and more accurate in their observation than the nurse who cannot. The nurse who can differentiate between the zone of thinking and the zone of fantasy is less likely to jump to conclusions about their observations or to make value-judgements based on prejudice rather than fact.

The study of each of the three zones can never be exhaustive. Each zone lends itself to further exploration. To explore Zone 1 is to explore the outer aspect of the self: our behaviour, speech and so on. It is also to explore the environment in which we live and move. It is to come to know more about the world around us.

To explore Zone 2 is similarly a potentially protracted process. There would seem to be no end to how much we can study our thought processes, feeling states and bodily sensations. Likewise examining our fantasy life can give us insights into the sorts of people we are and how we picture ourselves, others and the world around us.

All such exploration can be carried out either in isolation or in groups. If done in isolation, meditative techniques can be of value, and a selection of these are offered in the second section of this book. Often, however, the preference will be to conduct such exploration in groups. In this way we gain further insight through hearing other people's thoughts, feelings and observations and we can make comparisons between other people's experiences and our own. There are a variety of group formats—sensitivity groups, encounter groups, group therapy, training groups—in which to explore the self. Some of these are discussed in the next chapter.

After individual and group self-exploration, there is another approach, that of working in pairs. To explore the self in the company of one other person can be a rewarding and economical method. Economical in that the time available can be equally divided between the two people. Co-counselling can be a useful method based on the two-person format and this will be discussed as a method of self-awareness training.

Other methods of self-awareness training include the use of role-play, social skills training and assertiveness training. These are all well documented in the literature (see, for example, Alberti and Emmons, 1982 and Wilkinson and Canter, 1982), and courses in these forms of training are frequently organised by women's groups, growth centres and extra-mural departments of colleges and universities. In nurse education and training, the use of video and cassette players can enhance self-awareness, though taking part in their use should always be voluntary. No one should ever be forced to take part in a video-taping session. Such enforced self-awareness training is rarely valuable and may well cause embarrassment and self-consciousness for the shy individual.

Work on the body can be valuable in the field of awareness and thus Reichian bodywork, yoga, tai chi, the martial arts, gymnastics, sport and exercise all have their place as methods of self-awareness training. A quieter, reflective approach is through the written word: the keeping of diaries and journals can aid the awareness process and serve as a continuous historical document.

Probably the ideal is a combination of a variety of approaches: introspective, with a group, active and passive. In this way, the self is studied in all its aspects and no one aspect is developed at the expense of any other. The eclectic approach is healthier, in that it encourages the combination of sport and exercise with meditation or contemplation. It also allows for social relationships to develop alongside periods of solidarity. In short, it is a 'normal' and sociable process. If self-awareness training is to have a practical end—the enhancement of interpersonal relationships and skills—a balanced approach is vital.

Figure 1.4 maps out the wide variety of aspects of self-awareness and some of the methods that may be used in the development of such awareness. Note that it is not exhaustive of all possible aspects of self-awareness nor inclusive of all possible methods, nor is it a hierarchy: no aspect or method is more or less important than any other.

Possible aspects of self-awareness	Practical methods of developing aspects of self-awareness

1. Thoughts, including:
  (a) stream of consciousness
  (b) ideas
  (c) fantasy
  (d) delusions/false beliefs
  (e) recurrent thought patterns, etc.
	1. Discussion/conversation/group work
	2. Introspection
	3. Meditation
	4. Brainstorming exercises
	5. Co-counselling
	6. Writing
	7. Use of problem-solving strategies, etc.

2. Feelings, including:
  (a) anger
  (b) fear
  (c) grief
  (d) embarrassment
  (e) joy, happiness, etc.
	1. Discussion/conversation/group work
	2. Introspection
	3. Meditation
	4. Gestalt exercises
	5. Co-counselling
	6. Counselling/therapy
	7. Psychodrama
	8. Role-play
	9. Cathartic exercises
	10. Encounter/sensitivity training, etc.

3. Spirituality, including:
  (a) clarification of belief systems
  (b) life philosophy
  (c) awareness of choice of expression, of spiritual needs, etc.
	1. Discussion/conversation/group work
	2. Meditation
	3. Prayer
	4. Aesthetic experience (e.g. art, music, etc.)
	5. Reading
	6. Life-planning, etc.

4. Sensation, including:
  (a) taste
  (b) touch
  (c) smell
  (d) hearing
  (e) sight
  (f) kinaesthetic
  (g) proprioceptive, etc.
	1. Focussing attention on one or more sensation(s)
	2. Group exercises
	3. Use of sensory stimulation/deprivation
	4. Gestalt exercises, etc.

5. Sexuality, including:
  (a) orientation (heterosexual, homosexual, bisexual)
  (b) expression, etc.
	1. Discussion/conversation/group work
	2. Counselling/co-counselling
	3. Values, clarification exercises, etc.

Possible aspects of self-awareness	Practical methods of developing aspects of self-awareness

6. Physical status, including:
  (a) the body systems
  (b) status in terms of health/illness
  (c) the link between emotional and physical status, etc.
	1. Self examination
	2. Medical examination
	3. Autogenic training
	4. Exercise
	5. Yoga, Tai Chi, etc.
	6. Meditation
	7. Massage
	8. Alexander technique
	9. Reichian bodywork, etc.

7. Appearance, including:
  (a) dress
  (b) personal style
  (c) height, weight, etc.
	1. Discussion/conversation/group work
	2. Self and peer assessment
	3. Self-monitoring
	4. Video, etc.

8. Knowledge, including:
  (a) subjective, 'personal' knowledge
  (b) objective 'public' knowledge
  (c) gaps in knowledge, etc.
	1. Discussion/conversation/group work
	2. Examination/testing/quizzing
	3. Brainstorming
	4. Self- and peer-assessment
	5. Reading/studying
	6. Use of journals/diaries, etc.

9. Practical, interactive and technical skills, including:
  (a) listening skills
  (b) counselling skills
  (c) group skills
  (d) range of practical skills, etc.
	1. Discussion/conversation/group work
	2. Role play
	3. Video
	4. Social skills training exercises
	5. Counselling skills training exercises, etc.

10. Needs and wants, including:
  (a) financial/material
  (b) physical
  (c) love and belonging
  (d) achievement
  (e) knowledge
  (f) aesthetic
  (g) spiritual
  (h) self-actualisation, etc.
	1. Discussion/conversation group work
	2. Values clarification exercises
	3. Life style evaluation
	4. Brainstorming and use of problem-solving cycle, etc.

11. Dreams	1. Maintenance of dream journal 2. Dream analysis (e.g. gestalt, Jungian, etc.) etc.

Possible aspects of self-awareness	Practical methods of developing aspects of self-awareness

12. Verbal activity, including:
  (a) use of particular words or phrases
  (b) active and latent vocabulary
  (c) accent, pronunciation
  (d) use of silence, etc.
	1. See below, under 13.

13. Non-verbal activity, including:
  (a) facial expression
  (b) eye contact (gaze)
  (c) gestures
  (d) proximity to others
  (e) use of touch
  (f) body position/posture, etc.
	1. Discussion/conversation/group work
	2. Video
	3. Role play/psychodrama
	4. Self- and peer-assessment
	5. Use of mirrors
	6. 'Conscious use of self', etc.

14. Self, in relation to others, including:
  (a) feeling for others
  (b) ability to give attention
  (c) confidence/lack of confidence with others, etc.
	1. Discussion/conversation/group work
	2. Assertion training exercises
	3. Counselling training exercises
	4. Social skills training
	5. Co-counselling, etc.

15. Values, including:
  (a) values system
  (b) moral code
  (c) open/closed mindedness
  (d) areas of prejudice, etc.
	1. Discussion/conversation group work
	2. Values clarification exercises
	3. Use of rating scales, etc.

16. Unknown/undiscovered aspects, including:
  (a) subpersonalities
  (b) transpersonal aspects
  (c) unconscious aspects, etc.
	1. Self-disclosure
	2. Co-counselling
	3. Transactional analysis
	4. Self-analysis/psychoanalysis, etc.

Fig. 1.4 *Methods of developing self-awareness.*

Self-awareness and the nurse

Having discussed a concept of the self and examined some methods of developing self-awareness, we may now ask why the nurse should need to develop self-awareness.

In the first instance, to discover more about ourselves is to differentiate ourselves from others. We can discover the difference between our thoughts and feelings and the thoughts and feelings of those with whom we interact. This is an important issue. If we cannot make such a differentiation we may feel 'invaded' by others or be unable to determine the difference between ourselves and others. For example, if we are talking to someone who is severely depressed, we may find ourselves caught up in their depression and become upset ourselves. This is because we cannot differentiate between *that* person's feelings and our own. Self-awareness can enable us to clarify our own position with regard to others. Our ego-boundaries are strengthened and we do not feel the need either to take over other people or to be taken over by them. Our problems are our problems and other people's problems remain their own. Such differentiation is vital in areas such as psychiatric nursing, the care of the dying or intensive care, where real involvement is necessary. Real involvement paradoxically, requires of us the ability to remain outside the other person's problem. Otherwise we may be swallowed up and lost within their anguish and can be of little help to them.

To become more aware of ourselves is also to learn conscious, intentional use of ourselves. We become agents: we are able to act rather than feel acted upon. We learn to realise how we can use ourselves to the full benefit of ourselves and others. To have awareness of how we may act gives us a greater range of choices. If we are blind to many aspects of ourselves we are also blind to the possibilities open to us. Increased self-awareness brings increased personal choice.

Once we can combine these two aspects—differentiation from others and an increased awareness of the range of choices available to us—we can be more sensitive to the needs of others. Indeed, we can even choose to *forget ourselves* in order to give ourselves more completely to others. Note, however, that such forgetting of the self is done through *choice* rather than through being unaware.

These are all vital issues in the field of nursing. Requiring as it does close association with others and involvement with their thoughts, feelings and bodies, it is of paramount importance in nursing that we, as nurses, help others through the use of ourselves. Indeed, self-awareness training must be an integral part of interpersonal skills training. Counselling and group skills can only be undertaken alongside such self-development. Discussing emotional and practical issues with others requires the ability to set aside one's own personal problems. Otherwise we run the risk of projecting our own problems on to others. The mental mechanism 'projection' refers to our tendency to see in others qualities or problems that are, in fact our own, but of which we are unaware. As we get to know ourselves better, we cut down the likelihood of projection occurring. We learn to reown projections, to see others more clearly and as they *really* are, rather than as we *imagine* they are. We learn to become more objective in our dealings with others. This is not to argue for a cold, clinical distance between ourselves and our patients but to acknowledge that we cannot begin to help others to solve their own health or life problems until we can see the difference between *their* problems and our own.

Part Two of this book offers a series of simple exercises aimed at increasing self-awareness within the context of counselling and group work. This chapter has offered a clear model of the concept of self and a variety of methods of developing self-awareness, and has suggested some reasons why nurses need to develop such awareness.

Chapman and Gale (1982) note the curious paradox involved in developing self-knowledge or self-awareness. They note that to gain knowledge of something does not normally alter the thing itself. To know a chemical formula, for instance, does not cause that formula to change. In the case of self-awareness, however, the knowledge gained about self causes the self to change. Of course, we are complex creatures, not reducible to any particular theory or concept, and any concept of the development of self-awareness must be an over-simplification. Such theorising can only act as a guide or as a means of clarification. The rest is up to the individual reader.

It is worth repeating the point made at various stages throughout this chapter: that the aim of self-awareness training is to enable us to increase our interpersonal skills. Self-awareness should enable us to improve our ability to understand and communicate with others. The path to such awareness is, however, fraught with problems. First is the problem of egocentricity. It is possible to become caught up in the idea of understanding the self to the point of becoming self-indulgent, selfish or even solipsistic. (Solipsism is the belief that it is the individual who has created the world, or who is the centre of the universe.) Clearly, such positions are not compatible with the altruism or concern for others necessary to the nurse. Second, it is possible for those who develop self-awareness to believe that they have discovered insights that set them apart from others or even make them better people. A sign of such development is sometimes the loss of sense of humour—those who adopt the (false) sense of the 'wise person' can be notoriously humourless and earnest. True self-awareness more usually brings a sense of humility and awe at the sheer vastness of the task undertaken. To continue with that task is easier if a sense of humour is maintained and, particularly, the ability to laugh at oneself. For this reason the company of others in undertaking the task, the maintenance of a 'light' atmosphere and the ability to integrate the exploration of self with a wide variety of other pursuits is the best recipe for a programme of self-awareness development. The best awareness groups are invariably light-hearted affairs. Certainly, self-disclosure to others is best facilitated within a light-hearted atmosphere. Finally comes the issue of voluntariness. Self-awareness cannot be forced upon people. It must be a voluntary process. Nurse tutors, senior nurses and others who organise groups of this sort would do well to notice what Heron (1977b) calls the 'voluntary principle'. This is a principle invoked at the beginning of any self-awareness training course and repeated throughout such a course, to the effect that at no time will anyone have any pressure put upon them to take part in any exercises or activities except of their own free will. If self-awareness is about developing autonomy and becoming aware of choices, it is of paramount importance to ensure that such choices are exercised from day one. Accepting other people's frailties, their reserve, and their choice not to disclose aspects of themselves until they are ready, are all part of the process of facilitation in this field. Such understanding on the part of the facilitator, particularly in the early stages of courses, will do much to increase confidence and create an atmosphere conducive to self-understanding.

Recommended reading

Bond M. and Kilty J. (1982). *Practical Methods of Dealing with Stress*. Human Potential Research Project, University of Surrey, Guildford, Surrey.

Canfield J. and Wells H.C. (1976). *100 Ways to Enhance Self-Concept in the Classroom*. Englewood Cliffs, New Jersey: Prentice Hall.

Chapman A.J. and Gale A. (1982). *Psychology and People: A Tutorial Text*. London: The British Psychological Society and the Macmillan Press, Ltd.

Claus K.E. and Bailey J.T. (1980). *Living with Stress and Promoting Well-Being: A Handbook for Nurses*. St. Louis, Missouri: C.V. Mosby Co.

Ernst S. and Goodison L. (1981). *In Our Own Hands: A Book of Self-Help Therapy*. London: The Women's Press.

Ferruci P. (1982). *What We May Be*. Wellingborough: Turnstone Press.

Francis D. and Woodcock M. (1982). *Fifty Activities for Self-Development*. Aldershot: Gower Publishing Co. Ltd.

Heron J. (1977). *Catharsis in Human Development*. Human Potential Research Project, University of Surrey, Guildford, Surrey.

Jourard S.M. (1964). *The Transparent Self*. Princeton, New Jersey: Van Nostrand.

——(1977). *Self-Disclosure: An Experimental Analysis of the Transparent Self*. New York: Wiley Interscience: John Wiley & Sons.

Rogers C.R. (1967). *On Becoming a Person*. London: Constable.

——(1977). *On Personal Power*. London: Constable.

Shaffer J.B.P. (1978). *Humanistic Psychology*. New Jersey: Prentice Hall.

Stevens J.O. (1971). *Awareness: Exploring, Experimenting, Experiencing*. Moab, Utah: Real People Press.

CHAPTER TWO

The Concept of Experiential Learning

This chapter briefly explores the concept of experiential learning. It is not a treatise on the subject. Experiential learning theory has been explained elsewhere (Keeton *et al.*, 1976; Kolb, 1984). What is intended here is that the reader will gain insight into the nature of learning through experience.

The characteristics of experiential learning

We all learn through experience, whether directly, through taking action, through being involved in a situation, or by observing others. Every situation is an experiential learning situation. To define experiential learning in such broad terms would, however, be of little value. The concept would be so vast as to lose any meaning.

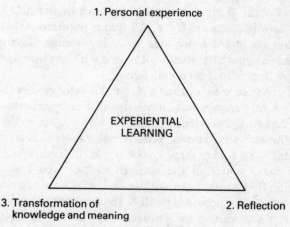

Fig. 2.1   *The concept of experiential learning.*

The concept of experiential learning involves the three elements identified in Figure 2.1.

First, the concept involves personal experience: the fact of something happening to us, or our being actively involved in a situation. Such experience involves the whole of us: our thinking, feeling, behaving and body sense. The concept of personal experience can be loosely defined as our involvement in a situation.

The second element of experiential learning is the process of reflection. Often after something has happened to us, we have reason to ponder on it but this is not *necessarily* the case. Things may happen to us that we either do not notice or we quickly dismiss. In experiential learning, however, the reflective process is vital. It is only through such reflection that we can ever achieve the third element: the transformation of knowledge.

Experiential learning differs from the more usual classroom methods by having a different view of the concept of knowledge. Many traditional methods merely offer the student pre-packaged knowledge in indigestible chunks, upon which no reflection takes place. It is as if the object of learning was to be filled with knowledge, which may, at a later date, be cashed in through examinations. Paulo Freire (1970, 1972) has referred to this as the 'banking' concept of education. Knowledge is fed into the student who reproduces it, usually unchanged, at a later date. Much traditional nurse education has been of this sort. Such an approach, apart from being fairly dull and unimaginative, presupposes a particular view of the nature of knowledge. From this traditional 'banking' point of view, knowledge is unchanging and constant. In other words, 'facts are facts'. All that is required is that the student takes on board more and more knowledge. The educated person or the educated nurse is the one who has managed to absorb more 'facts' than their colleagues.

An alternative view of the nature of knowledge sees the individual as a vital part of what knowledge is. Far from being external and unchanging, knowledge is relative and subject to the perception of the one who knows. Knowledge can be 'created' by the individual, who makes sense of the world around them. Such an account takes notice of the concept of 'personal knowledge'— knowledge that comes from within. Indeed, knowledge cannot be divorced from the person who does the knowing: they are bound together. 'Facts' cannot exist outside the person who knows them. The educated person or educated nurse is more than a person who collects facts: they are able to question, develop theories and make sense of their world from a personal point of view. Thus Freire argues for a 'problem-posing' approach to education. Rather than treating students as empty vessels to be filled with knowledge, he acknowledges that students bring to any learning situation a wealth of experience. It is the task of the educator to pose those students problems in order that they may question and re-evaluate their knowledge. Thus the nurse coming to the Introductory Course does so with a background of life experience and with a wide variety of beliefs, attitudes and theories. It is the tutor's task to help the student to re-evaluate those ideas and attitudes, not merely to *replace* them with a handed-down set of 'facts'. The tutor in this model is not the fount of knowledge, the one who can lay claim to the 'facts', but a fellow explorer who treats their students on an equal person-to-person basis. Carl Rogers (1983) uses the expression 'facilitator of learning' to describe such an educator.

Thus stages 2 and 3 of this model of experiential learning are its distinguishing features. Reflection on our experience, particularly if it is combined with discussion with others, can lead to our re-evaluation of what we know and understand. New meanings, new ideas emerge out of this reflection and pondering on personal experience.

Experiential learning is not, of course, to be viewed as a *replacement* for more traditional techniques; the *process* of experiential learning differs from more traditional methods, and a combination of traditional *and* experiential techniques can produce a powerful and comprehensive educational experience.

What then are the *methods* involved in experiential learning? Figure 2.2 lists the methods that are usually identified as experiential. All involve the three elements of personal experience, reflection and the transformation of knowledge.

Clearly, a number of these methods overlap and not all of them will be discussed in detail in this book. The recommended reading list at the end of this chapter contains books that give the procedures involved in all of them. All the methods can be used to enhance nursing skills in the context of interpersonal relationships. The focus of any learning in the school of nursing should be the nurses' personal life experiences and their ward experiences. Such a combination is vital fuel for the development of new and 'human' nursing knowledge.

Group discussions
One-to-one exercises
Role-play
Co-counselling and counselling exercises
Psychodrama
Simulation
Meditation
Relaxation exercises
Problem solving exercises
Structured exercises
Games
Guided fantasy

Fig. 2.2　*Examples of experiential learning methods.*

Learning through and learning from experience

Another way of understanding the concept of experiential learning is by the division of *learning through* experience and *learning from* experience (Burnard, 1983). In learning *through* experience, a situation is set up that may allow us to gain insight through participation. In learning *from* experience, we are required to look back at a past situation in our lives in order to glean new meaning from it or to compare it with our present situations. Both types of experiential situation may be set up by the individual working on their own or by the tutor working with a group of students. In the first instance (learning through experience), we may seek out an experience through which to learn. Such a process requires that we monitor ourselves throughout the experience and continuously reflect on our thoughts and feelings as we go. Alternatively, the nurse tutor may set up an experience from which a group can learn and afterwards suggest that the whole group reflects upon their experiences. In the second instance (learning from experience), the individual may systematically or randomly pick out past experiences on which to reflect and attempt to make sense of those experiences in terms of their present-day experience. Alternatively, the nurse tutor may invite a group to reflect on their past experience of a particular situation and jointly to draw conclusions from it. Such sharing of past experience can be a fruitful means of generating ideas for problem-solving and future planning. Figure 2.3 offers examples of situations for learning both through and from experience. Situations from the first column offer nurses the chance to explore *directly* what it may be like to be a patient. Reflection upon situations in the second column enable nurses to develop empathy with their patients, based on previous life-experience. Both routes to learning are powerful methods of understanding more directly the more subtle aspects of nursing care.

Learning THROUGH Experience	Learning FROM Experience
1. Taking other people's and having one's own blood pressure taken	1. Reflection on early childhood experiences
2. Sitting in a hospital out-patients' department	2. Recall of first experiences at school
3. Lying in a hospital bed	3. Discussion of hospital experience as a patient
4. Being fed by a colleague	4. Recall of being interviewed by a doctor
5. Being dressed by a colleague	5. Reflection on relationships with parents
6. Being lifted by colleagues	6. Recall of a specific happy incident from home life
7. Being blindfolded and led by a colleague	7. Discussion of past job experiences
8. Being washed by a colleague	8. Reflection on being male/female
9. Visiting the GP	9. Reflection on experience of bereavement
10. Running a discussion group	10. Recall of four formative experiences from life

Fig. 2.3   *Examples of situations for learning THROUGH and FROM experience.*

Finally, it is useful to identify the characteristics that consistently emerge from the theory and practice of experiential learning. These are as follows:

(a) There is an emphasis on action.
(b) Students are encouraged to reflect on their experience.
(c) A clarifying approach is adopted by the tutor.
(d) There is an accent on personal experience.
(e) Human experience is valued as a source of learning.

These characteristics are now examined in order to make sense of the concept of experiential learning.

There is an emphasis on action

Most experiential learning methods involve the participant in some form of action. This is not to say that they are 'doing something' in a trivial sense but that they are learning through the process of activity and movement. This can be viewed as the opposite of traditional teaching/learning strategies which require the learner to be passive and the teacher to be a dispenser of knowledge. Through activity we are engaged in learning through all our senses, not merely involved in some sort of thinking process.

Students are encouraged to reflect on their experience

Most writers in the field acknowledge that experience alone is not sufficient to ensure that learning takes place. Importance is placed on the integration of new experience with past experience through the process of reflection (Kolb, 1984; Kilty, 1982a; Freire, 1972). Reflection can be an introspective act in which the individual alone integrates new experiences with old. It can also be a group process whereby sense is made of an experience through group discussion. If reflection as a group activity is to be successful, the teacher is required to act as group facilitator and may require special skills and knowledge. The skills associated with group facilitation differ from the skills associated with the usual process of teaching, in that the group facilitator takes a non-directive and non-authoritative stance in relation to the students. In a reflective group, the teacher as facilitator neither ascribes meanings to experience nor offers explanations, but allows and encourages students to do these things for themselves.

A clarifying approach is adopted by the tutor

In the experiential approach, the teacher does not 'teach' in the traditional sense: he or she does not dispense knowledge or force *their* meanings onto the student's experience. Instead, the teacher helps the student to make sense of their *own* experience in their own way. After an exercise in which students practise counselling skills, the nurse tutor encourages quiet reflection on the exercise.

Rather than offering explanations for what the students have undergone, the tutor invites each student to comment on what happened and invites the group to 'make sense' of the exercise. The tutor may help the students to verbalise their feelings and ideas but does not attempt to direct them.

This is not easy! Teachers, perhaps by nature, like telling students about their own particular experiences or theories. To stand back and to allow personal discovery in this way is often to go against the traditional role of the teacher.

Through this process of clarification, nurses may develop an ability to trust their own judgement and to accept their own ideas and feelings. They no longer have to defer to the tutor but appreciate the value of their own thoughts about their experiences, both in the school of nursing and in the wards. In this sense, the tutor is acting as a true 'facilitator of learning'. In the literature on experiential learning, the term 'facilitator' is often used in preference to the terms teacher, tutor or lecturer.

There is an accent on personal experience

As long ago as 1932, Alfred North Whitehead discussed the problem of 'dead' knowledge and, using colourful language, asserted that knowledge kept no better than fish! (Whitehead, 1932). Experiential learning emphasises the evolving, dynamic nature of knowledge. Rather than viewing knowledge as fixed and unchanging, it stresses the importance of the student understanding and creating a view of the world in that student's own terms. Knowledge, then, is not something that is 'tacked on' to the person, it becomes part of the person themselves. What we learn changes our world view and changes us. This is what is to be understood by the accent on personal experience.

As a nurse continues through their training, what they learn becomes part of them. The nurse who becomes skilled at discussing problems with clients or patients changes as a result: the very personal experience of developing human skills helps the nurse towards an enhanced self-concept.

Human experience is valued as a source of learning

As we have seen, the accent in experiential learning, through its variety of techniques, is on experience. Malcolm Knowles (1978) stresses the importance of experience in the field of adult learning.

He maintains that as an individual matures they accumulate an expanding reservoir of experience that causes that person to become a rich resource for learning. Knowles argues that the resource should be tapped in the educational process because that reservoir of experience constitutes what that person *is*. Thus, for Knowles, an adult's experience is not something exterior but an integral part of that person's self-concept. Experiential learning is about human experience and it is human experience that makes us the people that we are.

Finally, it can be seen that what is under consideration here is (a) a learning method, and (b) an *attitude* towards learning. It is, therefore, a description of how to act in the educational process and also a model of education that stresses autonomous judgement, freedom of thought and the value of personal experience. In this latter respect it closely matches the process of nursing. If nursing is concerned with encouraging independence and autonomy, it is right that the procedures that are used in training nurses should reflect those qualities. Nurses who are trained to reflect on their experience, to form their own judgements and to develop a positive self-concept will be more likely to be in a position to encourage those qualities in their patients.

The development of experiential learning methods

Experiential learning methods have evolved from two sources. One is from the theorising of the American philosopher, John Dewey. Dewey believed that all educational processes should be based upon the life experiences of the students, and that school experiences and life experiences should be directly linked in a planned programme. Dewey was the founder of the 'progressive' school of educational thought as opposed to the 'traditional' school which stresses the importance of academic disciplines and the impartiality of knowledge. In stressing the importance of life experience as the foundation for the learning process, Dewey anticipated the work of Carl Rogers, Malcolm Knowles and other writers who democratised and personalised learning theory. His emphasis on practicality, the value of experience and the use of the students' own theorising, makes him a key figure in the history of experiential theory (Dewey, 1966, 1958, 1971).

The second source from which experiential methods are derived is the school of humanistic psychology. Humanistic psychology developed as a 'third force' in psychology in the 1950s and 1960s. The two other forces were behaviourism, on the one hand, and psychoanalysis, on the other. Humanistic psychology attacked behaviourism on the ground that it was an oversimplification of human experience and tended to treat the person as a very complicated machine. Psychoanalytical theory was seen as being over-deterministic. (A deterministic theory is one that sees present events as necessarily caused by past events.) Humanistic psychology opposed such determinism, arguing for the importance of human choice and free will. In other words, the person was not 'acted upon' by their past but able to make decisions about their life based on choice.

Thus behaviourism saw people as highly complex machines who could be 'programmed' or subject to positive and negative reinforcement. Psychoanalytic theory saw people as controlled by, and acting out of, their past. Humanistic theory, drawing from existential philosophy, saw people as free decision makers who could, and usually did, change according to their own wishes. Humanistic psychology was, therefore, an optimistic approach to an understanding of the person.

Humanistic psychology has as its central focus the person. It acknowledges that people are complex, individual and ever-changing. Thus no *one* theory of how people 'work' would explain *this* person in *this* situation. Humanistic psychology makes allowance for this variety of human experience. It places great importance on how the individual interprets their world and does not seek to develop a 'grand model' of how human beings develop, think, feel and act. Again, this is at some variance with behaviourism and psychoanalysis, as both offer overall pictures of how human beings are.

This theme of individual, subjective interpretation of experience underpins the thinking behind the exercises in Part Two of this book. Those exercises do not tell the individual what to expect or what they *should* experience: the emphasis is on the people involved discussing what happened to them as individual people with a wide variety of thoughts and feelings, beliefs and attitudes.

Again, the literature on humanistic psychology is vast (see, for example: Shaffer, 1978; Maslow, 1972; Rogers, 1977) and the pros and cons of this approach to psychology will not be discussed

here. Suffice to say that humanistic psychology has greatly affected both nursing and education. Carl Rogers's client-centred
counselling (Rogers, 1967, 1983) has revolutionised the approach
to nurse/patient interactions in psychiatric hospitals. This approach gave back to the patient their autonomy and self-direction. It was no longer the nurses who made all the decisions, but
the patients themselves. The humanistic theme has been carried
into the 1982 revised syllabus of training for ·psychiatric nurses,
and into the planning of the revised syllabus for mental handicap
nurses. It will also figure in the general nurse syllabus when that is
reviewed and revised.

The nursing process and the development of other nursing
models also offer evidence of the impact of humanism on nursing. These nursing models place the patient at the centre of the
nursing profession and emphasise the need for individualised care
planning.

In this section, a number of humanistic themes and approaches
are examined—for two reasons. First, the examination of these
themes helps to understand further the concepts both of self-
awareness and of experiential learning. Second, the themes under
discussion are often the original sources of the exercises offered in
Part Two of this book. Once again, the recurring themes will be
the importance of individual interpretation of experience, the process of reflection, and the value of discussion and sharing of experience.

Co-counselling

Co-counselling is a two-way process in which two people take it in
turns to spend time as 'counsellor' and 'client'. The client takes
time to verbalise and talk through issues and problems from everyday life, while the counsellor gives them attention. The counsellor in this relationship does not act in the traditional counselling
manner. In other words, they do not offer advice or attempt to
'sort out' the client. In this self-directed approach, the client him-
or herself learns to examine his or her own problems and to 'coun-
sel him- or herself', as it were. Each individual normally spends
approximately one hour in the role of counsellor and one hour in
the role of client. In this way, true interdependence is developed.
Neither party is wholly dependent upon the other. Responsi-

bility is shared, though responsibility for working through problems remains firmly with the client. The counsellor may be invited to make interventions at the request of the client, according to a pre-determined contract established between them.

Co-counselling can be used in a variety of ways. It can be a means of de-stressing for nurses working in areas of high emotional involvement. The very process of verbalising pent-up feelings to another person in an understanding and confidential atmosphere can be very therapeutic. Co-counselling can also be used as a means of developing self-awareness through the process of exploring inner thoughts and feelings and particularly buried emotion, in the presence of another person. It can also be used as a means of practical problem-solving, of talking out personal problems and making decisions about any aspects of the person's life.

Co-counselling developed in the USA under the influence of Harvey Jackins (Jackins, 1965, 1970) and, in this country, John Heron (Heron, 1974b, 1978). It has made its mark within the field of experiential learning. David Potts (in Boud, 1981) has described its use as a learning tool in a university course and James Kilty (1982a) has suggested the use of co-counselling in student nurse training. It can be a valuable aid to nurses wishing to develop greater self-awareness, and of particular value as a self- and peer-support system for nurses working in environments that are particularly stressful: intensive care units, children's wards, oncology departments, psychiatric units, and so forth.

Co-counselling training usually takes place through a forty-hour training course, during the course of one week, over two weekends or through a series of evening classes. Advanced co-counselling and co-counselling teacher training courses are also organised in colleges and university extra-mural departments.

Figure 2.4 is a simplified map of the theory behind co-counselling. This is a simple guide to the theory and practice of co-counselling and the reader is directed to the recommended reading at the end of the chapter for a more thorough explanation of what is involved.

The assumptions behind co-counselling are that people are potentially autonomous and able to exercise choice. Through the process of living, the individual experiences various types of stress which cause the blocking or repression of emotions. If those blocked emotions can be freed, then the person can once again be capable of making life-decisions and exercising freedom of choice.

1. People are potentially autonomous, self-directing, positive and able to exercise freedom of choice

↓

2. *HOWEVER* people are subject to a variety of stresses throughout life: early childhood experiences, partings, bereavements, difficulties in relationships, spiritual doubts and so forth

↓

3. Such stresses cause emotions (e.g. fear, anger, grief, embarrassment) to become 'bottled up' or repressed

↓

4. Through talking out and through emotional release (trembling, angry sounds, crying, laughter) those pent-up emotions may be released

↓

5. Such release generates insight and enables the person to think more clearly, to become less rigid, more autonomous and more able to take charge of their lives. They feel less 'acted upon' and more able to exercise choice. They can be spontaneous, positive and life asserting

↓

6. Co-counselling training, through working in pairs, offers people training in:
   (a) listening to and giving attention to others
   (b) reviewing and re-evaluating life experiences to date
   (c) the release of pent up emotion (catharsis)
   (d) handling other people's catharsis
   (e) problem-solving and life-planning skills

Fig. 2.4　*A simple map of the theory of co-counselling.*

Co-counselling aims at enabling the individual to express that blocked feeling and thus become more able to organise and take charge of their life.

There are implications, here, for nursing practice. As a general rule we want to calm people who are frightened, reassure those who are crying and stop people from expressing anger. Could we as nurses be trained to *enable* people to express those emotions as a therapeutic human act? In the fields of psychiatric and mental handicap nursing, the value of such an approach is perhaps clear: expressed emotion is presumably better than repressed emotion. It is also of value in general nursing. Post- and pre-operative situations, before and after childbirth, following bereavement: all these situations involve emotional experiences. Nurses can be trained to help their patients to express those feelings freely rather than (a) prematurely stopping them, or (b) feeling inadequate and unable to cope. Co-counselling offers one approach to coping with emotion. First, it enables the individual to experience their own emotional feelings and second, it trains people in handling other people's emotional release.

Co-counselling is a clear example of experiential learning in that it asks the individual to review past and present experience and to reconstruct their understanding in the light of the discoveries made. The co-counselling format is simple and can be readily adapted to a variety of learning situations in nurse education. A number of the exercises in Part Two of this book have developed out of co-counselling training.

Gestalt therapy

'Gestalt' is a German word for which there is no absolute English translation. It roughly means whole, integrated or complete. Gestalt therapy, an important influence in the humanistic approach to experiential learning, is a true mind/body therapy, aiming to integrate both aspects of the person. This it does by helping the individual to become aware of both psychological and physiological events as they happen. It thus has a 'here-and-now' focus. Gestalt therapy is only interested in the individual's past in as much as it affects their present-moment awareness.

Fritz Perls (Perls, 1969a, 1969b), a psychoanalyst, developed this approach to therapy, drawing from psychoanalysis itself, Reichian character analysis theory, existential philosophy and Eastern philosophy. It draws from psychoanalysis many beliefs about 'unconscious' or unrecognised factors at work in our minds and bodies. It develops Reich's (1949) work on the concept of emotion being trapped in sets of muscles and his emphasis on the need to recognise how we convey our psychological status through our bodies. It is an existential approach in that it encourages the individual to take full responsibility for themselves and for what they do, and acknowledges that it is *we* as individuals who invest our lives with meaning. Finally it borrows from Eastern philosophy a fascination with paradox: the existence of two apparent opposite states at the same time. Thus, it is paradoxical that as we learn, we realise our ignorance; it is a paradox that we can love someone and have very strong negative feelings for them.

Perls' gestalt therapy combined all these influences to create a type of therapy that *encouraged* feelings rather than resisted them. In many other therapies, for instance, the client or patient would be helped to oppose their feelings; thus the anxious person would be helped to relax. Perls' method was to encourage the person to *experience* their anxiety and, if necessary, increase it. Paradoxically, as this happened the person very often relaxed and felt more comfortable. It was through the acceptance of and experience of the emotion that release of symptoms came. Perls maintained that it is not until we fully accept ourselves as we *are* (and not as we would wish to be) that change can come about. Further, he noted that we often blamed others for our predicament ('my mother is a lot to blame for my condition'), or we appealed to some dubious theory about the nature of our make up ('I can't help it—it's the way I'm made!'). Gestalt therapy aims at helping the individual to experience and to *own* their experiences.

As with many humanistic therapies, gestalt therapy tends to use the following 'ground rules' during practice. Gestalt therapists usually prefer their clients to:

(a) Use 'I', rather than 'you', 'we' or 'people'. (Thus: 'I am unhappy at the moment', rather than 'you tend to get unhappy at times like this'.)

(b) Talk to others directly in the 'first person', rather than indirectly. (Thus: 'I don't agree with what you are saying', rather than, 'I didn't agree with what Peter said'.)

(c) Avoid asking questions, particularly 'why' questions. It is better perhaps to listen for the statement behind the question. (Thus: 'I am hurt by what you say', rather than, 'why are you saying that?')

(d) As far as possible, remain in the present rather than slipping into reminiscences. Gestalt therapists acknowledge that, in a sense, the 'present' is all there is. If we do not stay in the present, we are not fully awake to what is happening.

These 'ground rules' are valuable in helping the individual and group of people to remain fully in the present, to take responsibility for their thoughts, feelings and actions and to gain insight into themselves. As we shall see in Part Two of this book, they can be used as means of gaining insight into a variety of aspects of interpersonal behaviour.

The gestalt therapist works by helping the client to become more aware—aware of verbal expressions, tones of voice, body movements, gestures and so forth. Such a therapist does not interpret or offer explanations of what the client is saying but encourages the client to verbalise their own insights. The aim of the therapy is thus to increase self-awareness and self-understanding through moment-to-moment observation. It encourages the person to take full responsibility for themselves, to realise that, as 'authors' of their own lives they are free to exercise choice. In this respect, the gestalt process is similar to the co-counselling process. Both are non-interpretative and both emphasise the freedom of the individual.

The gestalt approach offers the nurse an alternative method of supporting patients. If the nurse can *allow* the patient to experience feelings—anxiety, unhappiness, loneliness as well as more positive feelings—then (according to gestalt theory) those feelings may change. As with co-counselling theory, this approach asks the nurse to accept the patient's feelings as they stand, rather than fighting them or trying to persuade the patient that they should feel otherwise. As with co-counselling, the model is that of experiential learning: learning through direct personal experience.

Used skilfully, gestalt therapy is an arresting, often oblique form of dialogue which involves a wide range of techniques. Perhaps the best way to try to capture something of its variety and range is through the use of an imaginary gestalt session. In the following exchange, a nurse, Jane, is talking to a patient, David, who has been admitted to an acute psychiatric unit because of his inability to cope with feelings of helplessness.

Jane: 'Tell me about things at home.'
David: 'There's nothing to tell really . . .'

Jane: 'Can you contradict that?'
David: 'There's *lots* to tell. . . . Yes, of course that's true!'
Jane: 'You're moving your arm in a sweeping gesture.'
David: 'Yes, it reminds me of the way my father waves his arms around when he's angry.'
Jane: 'What would you say to your father if he was here now?'
David: 'I'd say, You're always angry with me—you've never got time to talk.'
Jane: 'What's your father saying back to you?'
David: 'He's saying, you should grow up a bit and act your age!'
Jane: 'You're smiling!'
David: 'Yes, I realised that there is something in what he says!'
Jane: 'How are you feeling now?'
David: 'Sad, I suppose . . . no . . . angry, I'm angry with my father.'
Jane: 'Imagine your anger was sitting in that chair over there . . . what would you say to it?'
David: 'What a strange thing to ask! I'd say, why don't you leave me alone and stop messing my life up?'
Jane: 'And what does your anger say?'
David: 'You never let me out . . . I never see the light of day!'
Jane: 'What are you thinking?'
David: 'I never realised before how angry I really am—with my parents—with the whole family . . . mmm . . .'

And so the conversation continues with the nurse picking up the verbal and non-verbal cues that the patient is making explicit. No attempt is made by the nurse to interpret what David is saying but, left to his own devices, he makes sense of his own experience in his own way. This imaginary conversation cannot capture the element of surprise and often relief that can occur with this type of approach. Clearly too, training in gestalt methods is required and training courses of various lengths are held in different parts of the country. Whilst the example is from a psychiatric hospital, the techniques can be used in any hospital or community setting; with anxious patients for example, or those who appear to be 'stuck' with a problem or feeling. Gestalt methods can encourage new ways of looking at problems as well as enabling the generation of possible solutions.

Role-play

The use of role-play is fairly widespread in nurse education. It relates directly to psychodrama. Psychodrama was devised by a

Viennese psychiatrist, Jacob Moreno, who advocated the use of dramatic representations of painful, interpersonal events, played out on a stage (Moreno, 1959, 1969, 1977). His new method of therapy enabled people to try out new ways of behaving, to say things that needed saying but which in 'real life' were not said. In this way, the person was able to rehearse new approaches to life, to try things out, to experiment. Moreno was careful to make the psychodrama realistic and even went as far as designing and building a theatre in which the psychodrama took place!

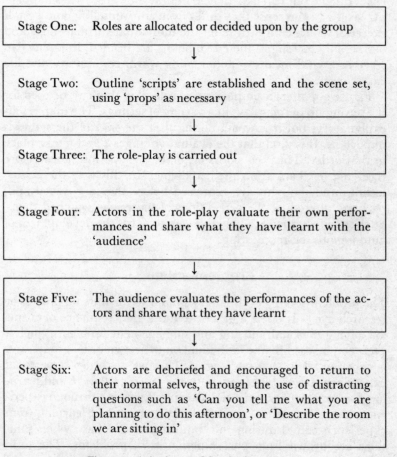

Fig. 2.5 *A simple map of the role-play experience.*

Role-play as an educational method emerged from this background. It is now fairly commonplace for tutors to set up situations in the classroom in which students are required to act the part of patients, doctors or other nursing staff. There is, however, an important issue here, which differentiates role-play from other types of experiential approaches. In role-play, students are acting a part; they are playing someone that they are not. Two important points must be made. First, it is vital that a de-briefing period is allowed following a role-play. In such a period students are encouraged to re-enter their own world, to return to the person that they are in real life. The second point is that role-play experiences differ from real experiences in that they are always happening 'as if'. In this sense they differ from co-counselling and gestalt exercises which concentrate on the individual's true feelings and on real life. As long as these two points are heeded, role-play can serve as a vital means of anticipating ward, community and life experiences.

Figure 2.5 offers a simple map of role-play that can be used for the setting up of role-plays in a variety of settings. The map is self-explanatory, but it is worth noting that the *order* of the stages is important. It is vital that the evaluative stages 4 and 5 take place in that order. Thus the actors evaluate their performance before receiving feedback from their audience. In this way the actors' feelings and thoughts are expressed before they are mixed and, perhaps, altered by the perceptions of those who watched them. Such self-evaluation is a valuable step towards the development of autonomous self-monitoring.

Problem-solving

The problem-solving cycle is very similar to the nursing process or research cycle. It offers a practical and logical sequence of events for solving personal, nursing and management problems. Such a cycle can be used by the individual on their own or by groups and is experiential in that once again it draws upon direct personal experience. It combines too, both the learning *through* and learning *from* aspects of experiential learning. Learning through experience comes as a result of using the cycle itself and learning from experience comes during the 'brainstorming' phase when solutions are drawn from past experiences of problems. The term 'brainstorming' refers to the free and spontaneous generation of

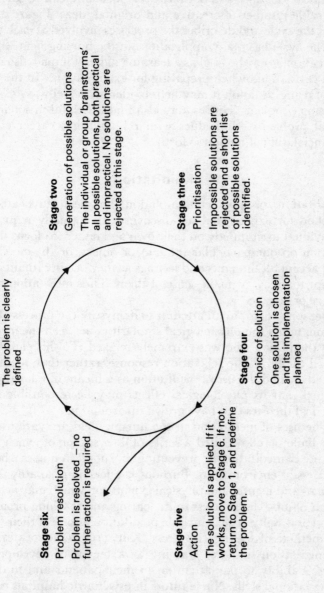

Stage one
Problem identification
The problem is clearly defined

Stage two
Generation of possible solutions
The individual or group 'brainstorms' all possible solutions, both practical and impractical. No solutions are rejected at this stage.

Stage three
Prioritisation
Impossible solutions are rejected and a short list of possible solutions identified.

Stage four
Choice of solution
One solution is chosen and its implementation planned

Stage five
Action
The solution is applied. If it works, move to Stage 6. If not, return to Stage 1, and redefine the problem.

Stage six
Problem resolution
Problem is resolved – no further action is required

Fig. 2.6 *A problem-solving cycle.*

ideas without any attempt at censoring or filtering out less than practical ideas. It does not rely upon logic and can release a considerable number of creative and original ideas. Figure 2.6 outlines the cycle and describes the processes involved at each stage.

The cycle has many applications in the nursing field. In nurse education it may be used as a learning aid and it may also be used as a revision aid when preparing for examinations. In the practical nursing situation it may help to identify novel·ways of solving nursing problems. Nurses may also find it helpful in solving personal problems—difficulties with relationships, career changes, financial difficulties and so forth.

Meditation

Meditation, or quiet contemplation, has been advocated as a method for experiential self-discovery. It normally requires the individual to sit quietly on their own and either (a) focus their attention on one particular thought or object, or (b) merely note and accept all thoughts and feelings as they occur without any attempt to follow or make sense of them. Thus meditation may be active or passive.

Benson (1976), in an attempt to demystify the process of meditation, noted the physiological similarities between the meditator and the person who was extremely relaxed. To this end, he preferred the term 'the relaxation response' rather than meditation. He advocated the use of meditation as a means of relaxation and argued that its physiological effects may be responsible for the mystical theories that have grown up around it.

The uses of meditation in the nursing field are various. Claus and Bailey (1980) edited a series of essays some of which discuss the use of meditation in preventing 'burnout' in nurses who work in stressful environments. Burnout is a feeling of apathy, dispiritedness and mental and physical exhaustion which may occur as a result of job-related stress in the caring and teaching professions. Bond and Kilty (1982) include meditation as one of their 'practical methods of dealing with stress'. Kilty (1982a) advocates the use of meditation in nurse training as a means of developing the nurse's ability to pay attention to their patients and to develop observational skills. Nurse tutors in psychiatric hospitals may use meditation (a) to help nurses to develop self-awareness and (b) to help nurses, and through them, their patients, to relax.

Meditation offers a rich and fruitful means of self-exploration and is a good experiential method of learning. It is best approached with an open mind backed up by a knowledge of possible explanations of the processes involved from the considerable literature on the subject. The recommended reading list at the end of the chapter includes titles on meditation and Part Two of this book includes some basic meditation procedures. Once learnt, such procedures can easily be taught to other colleagues and, where appropriate, to patients.

Meditation as a form of experiential learning differs from other approaches so far discussed in that it tends to be solitary and introspective. It can, however, take place in the presence of others and valuable learning can develop through the sharing of experience, as outlined in Figure 2.7. In working through the stages in

| Stage One: | The meditation technique is decided upon and, if necessary, taught |

↓

| Stage Two: | Individual members of the group meditate for periods of between 5 minutes and 20 minutes as decided beforehand |

↓

| Stage Three: | On completion of the meditation period each individual describes, comments upon or 'makes sense of' the experience to the group |

↓

| Stage Four: | The group discusses the collective experience with a view to developing a 'theory' about what happened |

↓

| Stage Five: | The stages from one to four may be repeated, as necessary, in order to test the theory |

Fig. 2.7 *Meditation as a group activity.*

this diagram, a form of 'experiential research' is taking place. Through the sharing of personal experience, the group as a collective is developing theories about that experience that can be further tested and refined.

Encounter groups

Although the term 'encounter group' has been used in a variety of ways (Smith, 1980), it is usually traced back to the 'T' or training groups of the social psychologist Kurt Lewin (Shaffer, 1978). Lewin's T-groups were not therapy groups but were designed instead to help managers and executives within large organisations to become more sensitive to the interpersonal and group-dynamic aspects of their work (Lewin, 1952). To provide an appropriate atmosphere for this sort of learning, the T-group leader worked at creating within the group a sense of openness, trust and emotional intensity.

The format of running intense, emotional small groups of this sort became popular with a wider clientele and developed, in the mid-60s, at the Esalen Institute, California, USA, and at the Center for Studies of the Person at La Jolla, California (Kirschenbaum, 1979). At the La Jolla centre, Carl Rogers developed his own style of non-directive or client-centred counselling in a group format (Rogers, 1970). He coined the term *basic encounter* to describe his particular version of the encounter group which stressed an unstructured, freewheeling approach in which group members were encouraged to develop and disclose their thoughts and feelings at their own pace. Rogers (who preferred the term 'facilitator' to 'leader') saw his role as one in which he created a warm, caring environment that was non-threatening and non-confronting. In line with his beliefs about the inherent ability of the person to develop and 'grow' at their own rate, he preferred not to use games, exercises or specific procedures for encouraging the development of the group but liked to allow it to evolve at its own rate. He asserted that he was always uncomfortable if he found himself resorting to 'techniques' and was happiest when he presented himself to the group in a spontaneous and completely natural manner (Rogers, 1977).

Whilst Rogers was developing his version of *basic* encounter, William Schutz, a charismatic figure of a different sort, was developing what he called *open encounter*, at the Esalen Institute, California (Schutz, 1967, 1971, 1973). Rather than just relying on group members to disclose thoughts and feelings spontaneously, Schutz used a variety of structured exercises. He combined ideas from psychodrama, gestalt therapy, physical exercises, oriental martial arts and meditation, to devise a potent new method of working with groups. Schutz's approach was much more *active* than Rogers' and he emphasised the value of physical as well as verbal activities. He attempted to heal the mind/body split by the use of exercises that provoked emotional release. Examples of such mind/body exercises can be found in Feldenkrais (1972) and Lowen and Lowen (1977).

Schutz also used a series of 'ground rules' similar to the ones in gestalt therapy. Schutz lists, amongst other things, the following rules:

(a) Be honest with everyone, including yourself.
(b) Pay close attention to your body.
(c) Concentrate on your feelings.
(d) Stay with the here-and-now.
(e) Take responsibility for yourself.
(f) Make statements rather than ask questions.
(g) Speak for yourself (use 'I', rather than 'you', 'we' or 'people').
(h) Speak directly to other people.

(Adapted from Schutz, 1973: 62–8)

Once again, all the familiar hallmarks of the humanistic approach to experiential learning are here: the personal responsibility, the accent on feelings and personal experience and the 'ownership' of those feelings and experiences.

The encounter group movement was limited largely to the United States and to the 1960s and 1970s, but the effects of that movement have been pervasive. The use of structured exercises in training situations is now widespread and most people will have participated in 'icebreaker' exercises if they have attended workshops and informal teaching sessions. The best-known series of publications that offer structured exercises in human relations training along the encounter group lines, are those edited by Pfeiffer and Jones (1974 and ongoing). Most of these exercises are adaptable for use in nurse training and the layout of the exercises is such that they can be conducted easily in a variety of settings.

Many other such compendia of encounter-format exercises have been published (see, for example: Lewis and Streitfield, 1971; Berger and Berger, 1972; Simon, Howe and Kirschenbaum, 1978; Canfield and Wells, 1976; and Francis and Young, 1979).

The structure exercise approach to experiential learning has been advocated by Marson (1979) as appropriate for the development of communication skills in nurses. Bailey (1983), writing of experiential learning techniques in psychiatric nurse training, argues that structured experiences can be useful in uncovering unconscious (or unknown) aspects of people's thoughts and feelings. He calls for the development of nurse tutors as skilled facilitators of such techniques.

These structured exercises can be of great value in the development of counselling and group skills in nurses. Through trying out new behaviours and by examining their thoughts and feelings in the supportive atmosphere of a group, nurses can develop more interpersonal confidence and a wide range of interpersonal skills. Such exercises should have a clear purpose. Many of the exercises in Part Two of this book are of the 'structured' variety and all are laid out in such a way as to make them readily usable in the classroom, in the ward, or in any other hospital or community setting. They have a clear and stated aim and are developed in a series which, as a whole, will help to develop a clear conceptual framework as well as increased interpersonal skills.

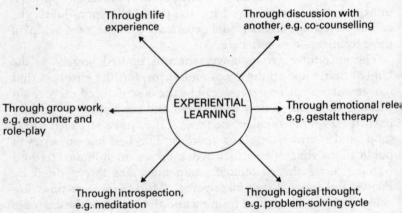

Fig. 2.8   *The varieties of approaches to experiential learning.*

The experiential learning approach: an overview

In the foregoing pages, a variety of approaches to the concept of experiential learning have been discussed. They vary in their focus and in their intention. What they all have in common is their use of human experience as the basis of learning. In the experiential model, learning is not a process by which facts are 'tacked on' to the person, nor is the individual 'filled with knowledge' as is sometimes the case in more traditional models. The experiential approach acknowledges the broad and vital nature of human experience and sees it as the potential medium for fruitful learning. Figure 2.8 shows the diversity of the approach by drawing together the examples so far discussed in the text.

Experiential learning and the nurse

The three important elements that go to make up the concept of experiential learning are personal experience, reflection and the transformation of knowledge. There are also at least three domains in which the nurse can benefit from the experiential approach to learning. These are personal growth, in general education and for the development of nursing skills (Figure 2.9).

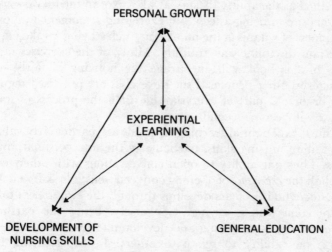

Fig. 2.9 *Experiential learning and the nurse.*

Experiential learning enhances personal growth by enabling us to develop self-awareness and to understand ourselves better. Through introspection and by receiving feedback from others, we can begin to piece together more and more of the separate parts that go to make up the complex whole that we are. Second, through such methods and particularly through the medium of group work, we can explore our relationships with others. As nursing is so particularly a profession involving relationships with others, it is crucial that we understand both ourselves and our abilities and weaknesses in our dealings with others. Once again, we cannot begin to understand those two facets until we begin to map the territory, until we become *aware* of what we are like and how we relate to others. Armed with such awareness we are better prepared to modify our interpersonal behaviour as we see fit.

Experience alone is not enough. What is being asked is that at regular intervals we *reflect* upon our experience and attempt to make sense of it. This sense of reflection can only come through self-training. It requires a certain discipline to stop every so often and look back at what has happened to us. In the normal course of events, much of our life experience passes by unremarked. It is here that the personal growth aspect marries up with this general education domain. As we develop greater self-awareness and greater sensitivity towards others, it is more likely that we *will* reflect upon what happens to us. Overall, what is required is what is described as the ability to 'stay awake'. Not in the literal sense, as an opposite to being asleep, but exercising a moment-to-moment awareness of what is going on. Again, such staying awake requires a certain discipline and training. Many of the exercises in Part Two of this book will encourage the noticing of fairly subtle changes in other people. If such exercises are practised regularly and become a part of everyday life then the process of staying awake will become second nature.

Third, experiential learning methods are particularly valuable in learning nursing skills, particularly the interpersonal, human skills. Thus our ability to open conversations with others comes through the *experience* of opening conversations; the skill in helping someone who is in tears develops through the *experience* of talking to someone who is crying. Conversely, being the partner of someone who is practising and developing such skills further develops our ability to relate to others. In experiencing being approached by another person and through experiencing the re-

lease of tears ourselves, we develop that most human of skills—
empathy. To empathise with another person is to 'stand in their
shoes', to understand intimately what it is to be that person.
Empathy is one of the most vital of all nursing qualities and must
be developed from the earliest days of nurse training. Empathy
cannot be learned through traditional teaching methods, lectur-
ing, project work and so forth. Experiential learning methods
offer the most direct means of developing the quality—a quality
that underpins all nursing skills, that is appropriate to and necessary for all nursing situations.

Part Two of the book offers the practical focus: a series of
planned exercises that demonstrate the theory so far in practical
terms.

Recommended reading

Boydel T. (1976). *Experiential Learning*. Manchester Monograph No. 5,
    Department of Adult and Higher Education, University of Man-
    chester.
Dewey J. (1938)/(1971). *Experience and Education*. New York: Dover Pub-
    lications.
Heron J. (1978). *Co-counselling Teachers Manual*. Human Potential Re-
    search Project, University of Surrey, Guildford.
Hewitt J. (1978). *Meditation*. Sevenoaks, Kent: Hodder & Stoughton.
Keeton M. and Associates (1976). *Experiential Learning*. San Francisco,
    California: Jossey Bass Pub.
Kilty J. (1982). *Experiential Learning*. Human Potential Research Project,
    University of Surrey, Guildford.
Kolb D.A. (1984). *Experiential Learning: Experience as the Source of Learning
    and Development*. New Jersey: Prentice Hall.
Perls F. (1969). *Gestalt Therapy Verbatim*. California: Real People Press,
    Lafayette.
Rogers C.R. (1970). *On Encounter Groups*. Harmondsworth: Pelican.
——(1983). *Freedom to Learn for the Eighties*. Columbus, Ohio: Charles E.
    Merril.
Schutz W.C. (1973)/(1982). *Elements of Encounter*. New York: Irvington
    Publishers Inc.
Simon S.B., Howe L.W. and Kirschenbaum H. (1978). *Values Clarifica-
    tion*. Revised Edition. New York: A. & W. Visual Library.
Smith E.W.L. (ed.) (1976). *The Growing Edge of Gestalt Therapy*. Secau-
    cus, New Jersey: The Citadel Press.

PART TWO

PART TWO

CHAPTER THREE

The Use of Experiential Exercises

The exercises in this section come under two headings: counselling skills exercises and group skills exercises. They are laid out in the following format for ease of identification and so that each exercise may easily be worked through in the practical situation:

1. Exercise no.
2. Aim of exercise
3. Group size
4. Time required
5. Materials and environment required
6. Process
7. Notes

For best results the exercises should be carried out exactly as described. After familiarity with a particular exercise has been gained, changes can be made to suit particular people or situations. The exercises should be carried out in a spirit of inquiry and approached with an open mind. The point will be lost if participants intentionally attempt to block what is happening in any way. To this end it is vital that participation is voluntary: no learning of any value can take place if participation is forced.

A useful procedure for planning the use of such exercises is outlined in Figure 3.1, an experiential learning plan.

In this cycle, a short theory-input is offered if the exercise is to be used in the classroom. (If it is to be used in a peer learning group, a discussion or reading period can be substituted for this stage.) Second, the concept and aim of the experiential exercise are introduced. Third, the exercise is carried out as outlined. Following the exercise, all participants feedback their experiences to each other as a group. Out of this feedback can be developed a fruitful discussion, and the learning that has taken place may become the basis for practical use in the 'real' nursing situation.

60

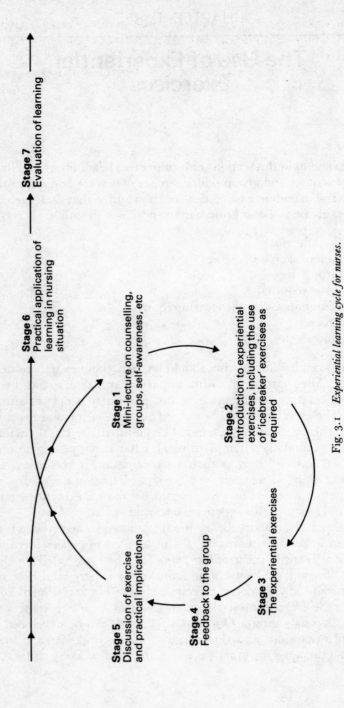

Fig. 3.1 *Experiential learning cycle for nurses.*

Stage 7
Evaluation of learning

Stage 6
Practical application of
learning in nursing
situation

Stage 1
Mini-lecture on counselling,
groups, self-awareness, etc

Stage 2
Introduction to experiential
exercises, including the use
of 'icebreaker' exercises as
required

Stage 3
The experiential exercises

Stage 4
Feedback to the group

Stage 5
Discussion of exercise
and practical implications

Finally, the learning is applied and the nurse carries his or her new skill or insight into the ward, community or other nursing environment. The experiential cycle can be evaluated through further discussion at a later date and further repetitions of the cycle carried out as required.

Stage one

The mini-lecture should be a short theoretical description of the particular topic being explored. The aim should be to create a theoretical 'scaffold' upon which the students can develop their ideas and experiences. If the exercises are being carried out by a group working on their own without a tutor, the aim is the same: to develop a simple theoretical model.

Stage two

The concept of experiential learning is introduced briefly and clearly. Any questions about the nature of the exercises are answered straightforwardly and students are offered the option of either taking part or observing their colleagues. Before the exercise is carried out, it is often valuable to use one or more 'icebreaker' exercises. 'Icebreakers' serve to create a relaxed and open atmosphere in which group members can enter more fully into the exercise being undertaken. A selection of such exercises will be described here: others may be found in a number of the publications listed under recommended reading at the end of this chapter. Most are lighthearted and should be treated as such.

Icebreakers similar to, or variants of, these exercises can be found in a variety of sources. (See, for example: Heron, 1973b; Pfeiffer and Jones, 1974; Kilty, 1982a.)

'Milling and pairing'

Group members stand and move around the room. At a signal from the facilitator they stop and pair off with their nearest colleague. The pairs spend a few minutes sharing thoughts on one of the following:

(a) A recent pleasant experience.
(b) Two interests away from work.
(c) Feelings about the group.

'Mad dog'

Group members stand and imagine that a mad dog is biting their ankle. Each member attempts to shake off the animal as actively (and noisily) as they can!

'Giant'

Group members move rapidly round the room with huge strides, imagining that they are three times their normal size. They may also make accompanying 'giant' sounds!

'Spot the squeeze'

A volunteer from the group stands in the middle of the group. The group members join hands. At a signal from the facilitator, a squeeze of the hand passes round the group. As a group member receives the squeeze, they must pass it on. The member in the middle attempts to spot the squeeze and identify the person passing it on. If they are successful, the person who was 'caught' becomes the person in the middle and attempts to spot the next squeeze.

'Alter ego'

Group members talk in the 'first person' as if they were another person in the group. Thus, they introduce themselves as that person and talk as though they were describing that person's thoughts and feelings.

'Push to the wall'

Members pair off, stand up and push against each others hands. At a signal from the facilitator they attempt to push their 'opponent' to the other side of the room.

'Yes and no'

The group divides into two rows, facing each other. One half shouts 'Yes' loudly at the other. The other half replies 'No' equally as loudly. The exchange continues ('Yes' ... 'No') and then at a signal from the facilitator the 'Yes' side changes tactics and shouts 'No', and the 'Noes', 'Yes'!

'A piece of music . . . a book . . .'

The facilitator asks each member in turn to describe themselves as follows:

(a) If you were a piece of music, what would you be? Describe yourself as that.

(b) If you were a book, what book would you be? Describe yourself.

(c) If you were a building, what would you be? Describe yourself.

Each group member is invited to imagine themselves as a different sort of object.

'Charades'

Each group member is invited to mime the title of a book, film, play, etc., in the manner of the party game Charades. The other group members guess what is being mimed.

'Hug'

Members of the group are invited to stand up and to hug each person in the room in turn.

'Mirroring'

Group members stroll around the room and periodically stop in front of each other. When they do so, each pair attempts to 'mirror' the body position and facial expression of the other.

'Sculpture'

Group members pair off. One member moves the other into any position that they choose, as a shop dummy might be moved. The group member being 'sculpted' stays in the position that their colleague designs for them. When all sculptures have been completed, the 'sculptors' wander round and 'mirror' other sculptures by standing in front of them and adopting their position.

'Chuckletum'

Group members arrange themselves on the floor with their heads on each other's stomachs. As soon as one person begins to chuckle, a ripple of laughter passes through the whole group.

'Numbers'

The group sits in a circle, holding hands. A message is passed round the group, using not words in the normal way, but numbers. Thus, an 'angry' message may be passed ('42', '18', accented heavily). Numbers change as the 'message' goes round but the tone remains the same. A second 'cheerful' message may then be passed with group members choosing new numbers said in a cheerful manner.

'Compliments'

Group members complete a 'round' in which they turn to the person on their left and complete the sentence: 'What I like most about you is . . .'.

'Awareness'

Group members complete a 'round' in which they turn to the person on their left and complete the sentence: 'Now I am aware of . . .'. They complete the sentence by noticing something about the person sitting on their left. Group members are encouraged not to rehearse their response but to respond spontaneously as their turn comes.

'Tug of war'

Group members line up in two equal groups. They stand behind each other and put their arms around the person in front of them. Each group faces the other. A chair or similar object is used as a 'rope' between the two groups and a 'tug of war' develops.

'Sitting sculpture'

One group member volunteers to walk round the group and 're-arrange' the people in the group in any way they choose. Thus, the volunteer may cross a person's legs or unfold their arms, etc. Various volunteers may take turns in rearranging the group in this way.

'Formative experiences'

Group members recall three positive experiences from their lives which they feel were formative and share those experiences with the group.

'Names'

Group members are invited to 'rename' members of the group or themselves. The facilitator should encourage the group to be tactful and use 'positive' new names! Group members may or may not want to explain why they choose particular names for particular people.

Clearly, some of these icebreakers will be easier to carry out than others. Much will depend upon how well group members know each other. If a lighthearted, open manner is adopted by the facilitator, most groups will find the exercises easy, amusing and sometimes revealing. Occasionally they may provoke stronger emotions and may produce hearty laughter or even tears. Such emotion is best accepted as it occurs *without* the facilitator either (a) too readily rushing to 'rescue' the group member, or (b) encouraging the member to leave the room. If emotional release is accepted in this way, a climate in which members can share feelings and experiences is more readily developed.

Two or three such icebreakers may be used to create an interested and participative atmosphere for the carrying out of the experiential exercises. As the group develops, and members get to know each other better and become used to experiential exercises, icebreakers may not be necessary and the exercise can be conducted 'cold'. It may be borne in mind, however, that icebreakers are often useful as a means of creating a break or a diversion in the middle of a series of experiential exercises. Used in this way, they can help to revitalise and re-energise a group during the course of a day's workshop.

Stage Three

In this stage, the experiential exercises described in the following pages are carried out.

Stage Four

Following the exercise, group members are invited to feedback their experiences of the exercises. Usually a broad open question, such as 'What happened?' will be sufficient to encourage people to share what happened during the exercise. It is important that each member is allowed to contribute and is 'heard'. This stage of the cycle should be as lengthy as is necessary to ensure that all that needs to be shared *is* shared. It is during this stage that the reflective process is at work and new learning is taking place through that reflection on experience.

Stage Five

During the fifth stage, new learning from the shared experience is applied in a practical way. Group members discuss the application of what has been learned to the ward or community nursing situation. Thus, if a counselling exercise has been carried out to develop listening skills, the group considers ways in which the nurses present could use their new listening ability to aid patient care. It is often useful if members undertake to try out a new skill the same day—away from the group. In this way the new learning is reinforced, becomes more real and is better remembered for the future. If new learnings remain in the classroom they are soon lost. If they are quickly carried out into the real world, they soon become part of the person's repertoire of behaviour. They are incorporated into the self-concept of that person.

This stage is vital. Experiential exercises on their own are insufficient. Stage five in the cycle serves as the bridge between the novel experience and the everyday experience. It is the stage in which self-awareness and self-development are consolidated to form practical human skills. Such development must be the aim of any experiential learning process in the education of nurses.

Stage Six

This stage, the stage of practical application, takes place away from the classroom or peer group. It is the stage in which theory is transformed into experience and in which the new human skills are practised. It is a time of trial and error, but also of discovery, as the nurse comes to realise the value of new-found self-awareness.

Self-monitoring is to be encouraged here and nurse tutors may wish to ask students to keep a journal of how they have made use of their newly developed skills. Such journals can be used for evaluation at a later date. They can also serve as a document of the progress of the individual's striving towards self-development and self-awareness. As such they map the progress and the pitfalls and can be valuable instruments for the design of future exercises and educational programmes.

It is essential that the nurse 'stays awake' during this stage, constantly noting his or her own behaviour, comparing it to the learning gleaned from the experiential exercises, and making modifications as required.

Stage Seven

Stage seven is the stage of the evaluation of both the experiential learning and the practical application of that learning. The following is a useful pattern for carrying out such an evaluation in a learning group.

1. Each group member gives feedback on (a) negative and (b) positive aspects of their performance. It is important that this order is observed so that the individual ends their own self-evaluation on a positive note.

2. The group member who has thus self-evaluated invites comments from the group and the tutor, again first on the negative aspects and second on the positive aspects of their performance.

This process incorporates both self- and peer-evaluation. Such a combination is valuable in that it encourages both reflection by the individual on their own performance and feedback from others. It is, perhaps, a more important form of evaluation than either a written report from a detached observer (e.g. the ward sister), or feedback from the tutor only. If such reports are required they can be combined *with* self and peer evaluation. In such a combination 'triangulation' has taken place: evaluative reports from three sources, as shown in Figure 3.2. In this 'triangulated' format, the individual nurse receives three types of evaluation: their own, their peers' and other professionals'. Such a format combines both subjective and objective types of evaluation and can of itself be a vital form of learning and a useful means of furthering self-awareness.

Continuing the cycle

Once a round of the cycle has been completed, the learning gained can be carried forward into a new cycle. Nurse training

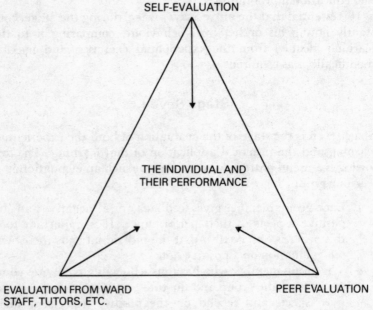

Fig. 3.2 *Triangulation in the evaluation process.*

programmes using a modular block scheme can incorporate the experiential learning cycle to create a continuous process of exercises, practical application of learning, and reflective evaluation. Such a scheme incorporates once again the three aspects of experiential learning identified in the previous chapter: experience, reflection and the transformation of knowledge and meaning.

The next chapters describe a series of experiential exercises that may be used to develop human skills: (a) in the one-to-one interpersonal relationship (counselling skills) and (b) in the one-to-group relationship (group skills).

The final chapter offers a number of exercises for the development of self-awareness that can enhance both counselling and group skills.

Recommended reading

Boud D. (ed.) (1981). *Developing Student Autonomy in Learning*. London: Kogan Page.

Francis D. and Young D. (1979). *Improving Work Groups: A Practical Manual for Team Building*. San Diego, California: University Associates.

Heron J. (1973). *Experiential Training Techniques*. Human Potential Research Project, University of Surrey, Guildford.

—— (1981). *Assessment*. Human Potential Research Project, University of Surrey, Guildford.

Kilty J. (1982). *Self and Peer Assessment: a Collection of Papers*. Human Potential Research Project, University of Surrey, Guildford.

Pfeiffer J.W. and Goodstein L.D. (1982). *The 1982 Annual for Facilitators, Trainers and Consultants*. San Diego, California: University Associates.

Pfeiffer J.W. and Jones J.E. (1974 and ongoing). *A Handbook of Structured Exercises for Human Relations Training*. Vols 1–ongoing. La Jolla, California: University Associates, Publishers and Consultants.

CHAPTER FOUR

Experiential Exercises for Human Skills: 1. Counselling Skills

An overview of the counselling process

Counselling is a therapeutic conversation between two people, in an understanding atmosphere. This definition is purposely broad, for, as has been discussed earlier, all the skills involved in the counselling process are also relevant to any nurse/patient relationship of any depth.

In this section, the skills involved in counselling are divided into (a) listening and attending and (b) counselling interventions. An intervention is anything that the counsellor *says* to the client. The exercises described here can be worked through systematically or particular exercises can be singled out to develop a particular skill.

In order to place these two groups of skills in context, a map of the counselling process is offered in Figure 4.1.

In stage one the counsellor and client meet, introduce themselves and slowly begin to get to know each other. This stage may be seen as paralleling the first stage of the nurse/patient relationship—the same processes are occurring. Carl Rogers (1967, 1983) notes that three clusters of qualities are necessary for the counsellor to function well in this stage: (a) warmth, transparency and genuineness, (b) empathic understanding and (c) unconditional positive regard. Warmth, transparency (or openness) and genuineness are self-explanatory: they are personal qualities that are necessary ingredients in *any* relationship. Empathic understanding refers to the ability of the counsellor to 'stand in the client's shoes', to imagine sensitively what it is like to be the other person. Unconditional positive regard is the quality of totally respecting the worth of the person—unconditional, because that respect is not dependent upon the *client's* feelings for the counsellor. The counsellor or nurse who has unconditional positive regard has genuine human compassion for others. Perhaps a simpler word for such a quality is love.

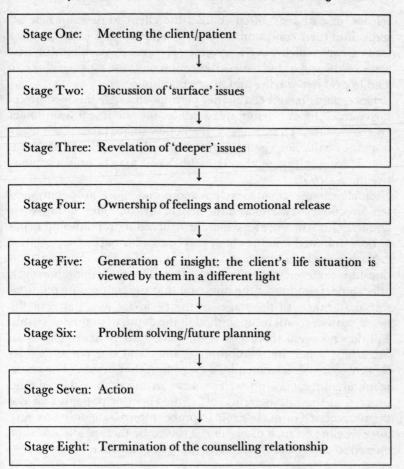

Fig. 4.1 *A map of the counselling process.*

As the counsellor/client or nurse/patient relationship develops, the client slowly tests the boundaries of the relationship through discussion of safe, 'surface' issues. Then, as trust develops, the topic slowly shifts to deeper existential issues. At this stage, the client often realises the true depth of feeling that they have about particular issues: emotional release may occur through the shedding of tears, the expression of anger or through embarrassed laughter. Such a release is known as catharsis and the counsellor or nurse can develop the skills required in helping a person through the process of cathartic release. Such emotional release, or catharsis, often enables the client to develop new insights into their condition. It is as though the tears or anger clear away a veil which covers possible solutions to problems or new ways of looking at life issues. Reflection on those new insights can lead to problem solving and future planning.

Once plans have been made, perhaps through the medium of the counselling or nursing relationship, the client will want to act on those plans. Thus, stage 7, the action stage, takes place away from the counsellor/client relationship and in the client's life situation. During this stage, the counsellor's role may be only a supportive one.

Finally as the client develops more and more autonomy and self-direction, they will need the help of the counsellor or nurse less and less. The time comes when the counselling relationship needs to be terminated and the client and counsellor part.

Such a cycle of events is an over-simplification. Human relationships are rarely as clear-cut as this. The cycle does, however, offer some signposts for the direction that the counselling relationship may take. All the stages in the cycle are also stages in the nurse/patient relationship, although the depth of that relationship will depend upon the needs of the particular patient. This is an important issue: the relationship is the client's or patient's relationship—it is determined by the needs of that person. The counsellor or nurse may do well to bear in mind that they should proceed at the rate determined by the client or patient. It is not the counsellor's or nurse's role to probe, interrogate or in any way force disclosure: such disclosure, if it is to be therapeutic, must be offered freely by the client and with their goodwill.

Listening and attending

To listen to another person is perhaps the most human of actions. In counselling it is the crucial skill. The experiential exercises that follow aim to develop the skills of listening and giving attention. Listening refers to the process of *hearing* what the client is saying. Such hearing encompasses not only the words that are being used but also the non-verbal aspects of the encounter. Thus *attending* refers to the counsellor's skill in paying attention to the client, in keeping attention focussed 'out', as described in the first chapter.

Throughout all the exercises in this chapter the words facilitator, counsellor and client are used for convenience. It should be noted that the words tutor, nurse and patient can just as easily be used in their place.

Once again, the participants must be exhorted to 'stay awake' during these exercises. It is vital that the person *notices*: notices their own feelings and thoughts, their own body position, posture, eye contact, etc., and also notices their partner in all these respects. The mystic, George Gurdjieff, maintained that for most of what we call the waking state, we were in fact 'asleep'—we simply did not *notice* (Reyner, 1984). The nurse who practises regularly the feat of such noticing becomes more observant, more sensitive towards the needs of others and more self-aware. Indeed, to notice in this way is to be fully present in the moment that is being lived.

The first series of exercises concentrate on a variety of aspects of listening and attending.

Exercise 1

Aim of exercise: To enable participants to get attention 'out'. **Group size:** Any multiples from 2 to a maximum of 20. **Time required:** Approximately 20 to 30 minutes. **Materials and/or environment required:** Large room or various small rooms; straight-backed chairs of equal height.

Process

1. The facilitator invites the group to divide into pairs.
2. Each pair nominates one of them as 'A' and one as 'B'.
3. 'A' describes in detail, for two minutes, what 'B' looks like: hair, facial expressions, clothing, etc. Such a description should be 'literal' and free of value-judgements.
4. 'B' listens impassively to 'A''s description.
5. After two minutes, the facilitator invites the pairs to exchange roles: thus 'B' describes, literally 'A''s appearance.
6. When both aspects of the exercise have been completed, the facilitator invites the group to reconvene and encourages feedback with an open question such as 'What happened?'
7. The facilitator makes no attempt to interpret what happened but may summarise the feelings and experiences of the group as appropriate.

Notes
Group members can be encouraged to use this method of paying
attention to and describing a person (or an object) outside themselves as a method of getting attention 'out' prior to talking to a
patient or commencing counselling. It can be done silently and
alone and is valuable as a means of freshening attention at any
time.

Exercise 2

Aim of exercise: To explore the verbal and non-verbal aspects
of listening. **Group size:** Any multiples from 2 up to a maximum
of 20. **Time required:** Approximately 40 minutes. **Materials
and/or environment required:** Large room or various small
rooms; straight-backed chairs of equal height.

Process
1. The facilitator invites the group to divide into pairs.
2. Each pair nominates one of them as 'A' and one as 'B'.
3. 'A' talks to 'B' for three minutes on one of the following topics:
   (a) interests away from work;
   (b) recent ward experiences;
   (c) past or future holidays.
4. Whilst 'A' is talking, 'B' does *NOT* listen.
5. After three minutes the facilitator invites the pairs to exchange
   roles: thus 'B' talks to 'A' and 'A' does not listen.
6. When both aspects of the exercise have been completed, the
   facilitator invites the group to reconvene and encourages feedback with an open question.
7. The facilitator makes no attempt to interpret what happened
   but may ask questions such as:
   'What was it like not to be listened to?';
   'How did you *know* that your partner was not listening?', etc.

Notes
A variant of this exercise is to have the pairs sitting back-to-back,
so that 'A' talks to 'B' but cannot see 'B'.

Following the experience of Exercise 2, it is common for a discussion to develop on the importance of non-verbal behaviour
when listening to another person. Egan (1982) offers a useful acro-

S —Sit *squarely*
O—maintain an *open* position
L —*lean* slightly forward
E —maintain steady *eye* contact
R—*relax*

Fig. 4.2   *The behavioural aspects of listening* (after Egan, 1982).

nym that aids the memorisation of the important aspects of non-verbal activity during the listening process. This is illustrated in Figure 4.2.

Sitting squarely means sitting directly opposite the person who is being listened to. An open position means that the listener does not have their arms or legs crossed; such crossings can create real or psychological barriers. Certainly, the closed position can convey a sense of defensiveness as we shall see in the following exercise. It is often helpful to lean slightly forward towards the client as this conveys a sense of interest in the person. Eye contact is of particular importance and should be steady, without any sense of glaring or staring. Finally, it is important that the listener should be, and should appear to be, relaxed. The listener who fidgets conveys a sense of impatience or, perhaps, lack of interest. Figures 4.3 and 4.4 illustrate two listening positions: an 'open' position and a 'closed' position.

These notes on the behavioural aspects of listening are offered as guidelines. Many of the non-verbal aspects of listening will be dependent upon the situation in which the client and counsellor find themselves. It is suggested, however, that the SOLER model offers a useful 'baseline' of behaviour from which to work. With it in mind, nurses can monitor their behaviour and, through such monitoring, enhance their self-awareness.

Exercise 3

Aim of exercise: To explore the verbal and non-verbal aspects of listening and giving attention. **Group size:** Any multiples from 2 to a maximum of 20. **Time required:** Approximately 40

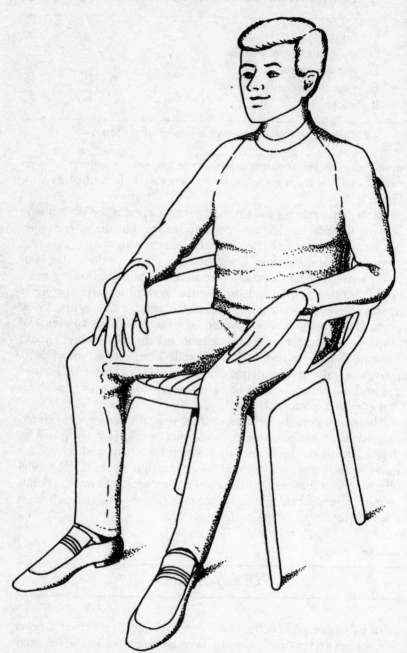

Fig. 4.3   *The 'open' position.*

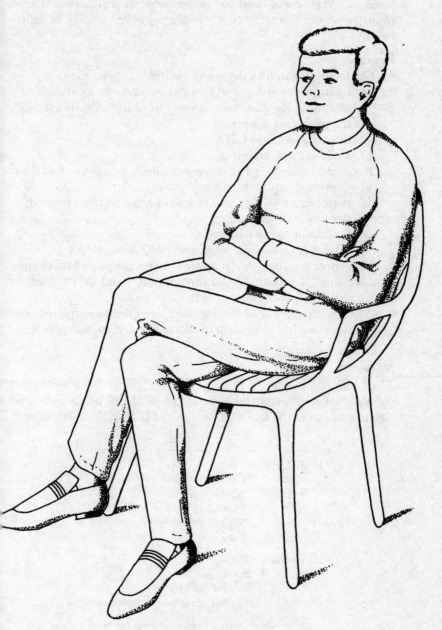

Fig. 4.4   The 'closed' position.

minutes. **Materials and/or environment required:** Large room or various small rooms; straight-backed chairs of equal height.

Process

1. The facilitator invites the group to divide into pairs.
2. Each pair nominates one of them as 'A' and one as 'B'.
3. 'A' talks to 'B' for three minutes on one of the following topics:
   (a) the problems of nursing;
   (b) music/books that I like;
   (c) student nurse training.
4. 'B' *contradicts* the SOLER behaviours described in the text thus:
   (a) does *not* sit squarely to the person;
   (b) maintains a 'closed' position with arms and legs crossed;
   (c) does *not* lean forward;
   (d) maintains *no* eye contact;
   (e) attempts *not* to appear relaxed *BUT listens to 'A'*!
5. After three minutes, the facilitator invites the pairs to exchange roles: thus 'B' talks to 'A' for three minutes and 'A' contradicts the SOLER behaviours but listens.
6. When both aspects of the exercise have been completed, the facilitator invites the group to reconvene and encourages feedback.

Notes

The facilitator is advised to suggest to the group that they do not overdramatise the contradiction of the SOLER behaviours and also to emphasise the fact that they are to LISTEN to each other.

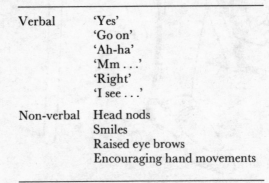

Verbal	'Yes' 'Go on' 'Ah-ha' 'Mm . . .' 'Right' 'I see . . .'
Non-verbal	Head nods Smiles Raised eye brows Encouraging hand movements

Fig. 4.5 *Examples of minimal prompts used in listening.*

An aid to the listening process is the use of 'minimal prompts', or noises that the listener makes to encourage the client to continue talking. They may also include head nods and facial expressions. Figure 4.5 offers examples of minimal prompts that are used in everyday conversation. The idea of identifying them is to enable the nurse to use them consciously and awarely out of choice rather than out of habit.

Exercise 4

Aim of exercise: To practise listening and giving attention with appropriate verbal and non-verbal behaviours. **Group size:** Any multiples from 2 to a maximum of 20. **Time required:** Approximately 40 minutes. **Materials and/or environment required:** Large room or various small rooms; straight-backed chairs of equal height.

Process
1. The facilitator invites the group to divide into pairs.
2. Each pair nominates one of them as 'A' and one as 'B'.
3. 'A' talks to 'B' for five minutes on one of the following topics:
   (a) the house/flat that I live in;
   (b) my family;
   (c) my hopes for the future;
   (d) any other topic.
4. 'B' listens to 'A' and observes the SOLER behaviours. Thus 'B':
   (a) sits squarely;
   (b) maintains an open position;
   (c) leans slightly forward;
   (d) maintains steady and comfortable eye contact;
   (e) relaxes.
   'B' may also use 'minimal prompts' as necessary but uses them sparingly.
5. After five minutes, the facilitator invites the pairs to exchange roles, thus 'B' talks to 'A' for five minutes and 'A' observes the SOLER behaviours and uses minimal prompts as necessary.

6. When both aspects of the exercise have been completed, the facilitator invites the group to reconvene and encourages feedback.

Notes
It is important that the facilitator emphasises that this is not a conversation. The listener should restrict themselves to minimal prompts only and not respond in any other way to anything that their partner says.

Exercise 5

Aim of exercise: To reinforce the skills of listening and attending with appropriate verbal and non-verbal behaviours. **Group size:** Any multiples from 2 to a maximum of 20. **Time required:** Approximately 1 to $1\frac{1}{2}$ hours. **Materials and/or environment required:** Large room or various small rooms; straight-backed chairs of equal height.

Process
1. The facilitator invites the group to divide into threes.
2. The threes are invited to nominate 'A', 'B' and 'C'.
3. 'A' talks to 'B' for four minutes on any topic.
4. 'B' listens to 'A', observing the SOLER behaviours in the text and using minimal prompts as required.
5. 'C' acts as process observer and makes notes on 'B's performance as a listener.
6. After four minutes each trio feeds back to itself in the following order:
   (a) the listener describes their own performance;
   (b) the client describes the listener's performance;
   (c) the process observer describes the listener's performance.
7. After ten minutes 'A', 'B' and 'C' exchange roles and conduct the exercise again.
8. When all participants have been in the roles of listener, client and process observer, the facilitator invites the group to reconvene and encourages feedback.

Notes

The trio's feedback in Item 6 above is vital. The order of the feedback encourages self-evaluation followed by peer-evaluation.

Exercise 6

Aim of exercise: To test the effectiveness of the listening and attending exercises. **Group size:** Any multiples from 2 to a maximum of 20. **Time required:** Approximately 1 to 1½ hours. **Materials and/or environment required:** Large room or various small rooms; straight-backed chairs of equal height.

Process

1. The facilitator invites the group to divide into pairs.
2. Each pair nominates one of them as 'A' and one as 'B'.
3. 'A' talks to 'B' for three periods of three minutes on any topic.
4. 'B' listens to 'A', observing the SOLER behaviours and using minimal prompts as required.
5. *Between* each three-minute period, 'B' paraphrases what 'A' has said, to 'A''s satisfaction. Then 'A' continues for second and then third periods of talking. The order is made clear in Figure 4.6.
6. After the cycle has been completed, 'A' and 'B' exchange roles and complete Stage 5 above.
7. When the entire cycle has been completed, the facilitator invites the group to reconvene, and encourages feedback.

---

1. 'A' talks to 'B' for 3 minutes.
2. 'B' paraphrases what 'A' has said.
3. 'A' talks to 'B' for a further 3 minutes.
4. 'B' paraphrases what 'A' has said.
5. 'A' talks to 'B' for a final 3 minutes.
6. 'B' paraphrases what 'A' has said.

Fig. 4.6 *Order of the exercise.*

Notes

This exercise can also be used with process observers. Such an observer can be allocated to each pair. Feedback in each trio would then take place as follows:

(a) the listener feedsback on their own performance;
(b) the client feedsback on the listener's performance;
(c) the process observer feedsback on the listener's performance.

Once again, such a procedure encourages self-evaluation followed by peer-evaluation and both can be valuable methods of enhancing self-monitoring and self-awareness. A form of this exercise was originally used by Carl Rogers (Kirschenbaum, 1979) as a method of non-directive counselling training.

Counselling interventions

The basis of effective human counselling is the skill of listening and giving attention. Second to this is the use of verbal intervention. A format for understanding the range of useful and therapeutic interventions has been devised by John Heron (1975b) and is called Six Category Intervention Analysis. The analysis offers six possible categories into which, it is maintained, all therapeutic interventions fall. A therapeutic intervention is one that enables the client to develop, to understand themselves further, or to problem-solve. The six categories that Heron identifies are shown in Figure 4.7, along with a brief description of each category.

What then, is the value of such an analysis of therapeutic interventions? First it identifies the *range* of possible interventions available to the nurse/counsellor. Very often in day-to-day interactions with others we stick to repetitive forms of conversation and response, simply because we are not aware that other options are available to us. This analysis identifies an exhaustive range of types of human intervention. Second, by identifying the sorts of interventions we use, we can act more precisely and with a greater sense of intention. The nurse/patient relationship thus becomes more precise and less haphazard: we know *what* we are saying and also *how* we are saying it. We have greater interpersonal choice. Third, the analysis offers an instrument for training. Once the categories have been identified, they can be used for students and others to identify their weaknesses and strengths. Nurses can, in this way, develop a wide and comprehensive range of interpersonal skills.

It is worth repeating that the skills identified in this chapter as counselling skills are exactly similar to the basic human skills used in day-to-day nurse/patient interaction. Thus an understanding of the full range of the six categories can enhance and enrich the quality of the nurse's approach to care. It should be noted too, that the analysis does not offer a mechanical approach to interpersonal skills training. The exercises here will not simply be a training in learning particular phrases or responses. The choice of words in any particular case is left to the individual student. The analysis indicates a *type* of response. This is an important issue. The choice of words, the tone of voice, the non-verbal aspects of a particular response must develop out of the individual's belief and value system and out of their life experience. Those aspects of the response are also dependent upon the situation at the time and upon the people involved. A mechanical, learning-by-heart approach to counselling or interpersonal skills would, therefore, be inappropriate. In the descriptions of the following exercises, examples are offered but when the exercises are carried out each student will have to find their own words, their own expressions, and their own personal approach; this affirms the true principle of human skills training—the honouring of personal experience developed through observation and reflection.

The category	What the counsellor/nurse does
1. Prescriptive	Makes suggestions, recommends behaviour to the client/patient.
2. Informative	Gives new knowledge or information to the client/patient.
3. Confronting	Challenges restrictive or repetitive attitudes, beliefs or behaviours of the client/patient.
4. Cathartic	Helps the client/patient to release tension through tears, trembling, angry sounds or laughter.
5. Catalytic	Helps draw out information from or encourages self-discovery in the client/patient.
6. Supportive	Affirms the worth of, is supportive of the client/patient.

Fig. 4.7   *The six categories of therapeutic intervention* (after Heron, 1975 and 1977b).

Two principles should be noted when using these exercises. Participation in them should be voluntary; growth in interpersonal development can never be enhanced if it is enforced—indeed such a concept may be a contradiction in terms. This then is the voluntary principle. The other principle is the gymnasium principle (Heron, 1977b). Just as a gymnast exercises in isolation one set of muscles that would not normally be used in that way in real life, so the following exercises highlight one particular aspect of the counselling/interpersonal relationship. In this respect, they may at times seem artificial. When combined with a full range of human responses, however, they make sense. The learning from a particular exercise needs to be incorporated into everyday life, just as gymnasts need to use all their muscles in everyday life.

Figure 4.8 offers some examples of what may constitute interventions in the six categories. It must be repeated, however, that the important issue is that such interventions develop naturally out of the context of the counsellor/client or nurse/patient interaction. The examples are offered as a means of clarifying the concept of the six category intervention analysis, not as exemplars or as 'ideal types' of intervention. In the real situation, the real choice of words that is used will depend upon the context; the aim of six category intervention analysis is to describe various *types* of interventions.

1. Prescriptive	1. 'Perhaps you would like to talk to your husband about this.'
	2. 'I suggest you tell the doctor about the rash.'
2. Informative	1. 'This medication may make you feel drowsy.'
	2. 'There is a Marriage Guidance Council Office in . . .'
3. Confronting	1. 'I notice that you very regularly use that expression.'
	2. 'We agreed to stop this meeting at 3 pm: we will stop now.'
4. Cathartic	1. 'It's all right by me if you feel you want to cry.'
	2. 'What do you *really* want to say to your mother?'
5. Catalytic	1. 'Can you tell me more?'
	2. 'You feel happy about that?'
	3. 'What did you do then?'
6. Supportive	1. 'I'm very pleased that things have worked out well for you.'
	2. 'I appreciate your being here.'

Fig. 4.8   *Some possible examples of interventions within the six categories.*

In a more general sense, the six categories of intervention have a wider application, beyond the counselling relationship. The nurse working in a hospice, for example, may need considerable cathartic skills in order to enable the expression of feelings; the ward sister/charge nurse will require prescriptive skills when delegating ward duties; all nurses require the ability to be appropriately supportive.

There may be situations in which skilful use of a *particular* category may be required in this way. The nurse who is skilled in all six categories can deftly select the appropriate category for the right situation. Figure 4.9 offers some examples of nursing situations in which one particular category may be used more. They can *only* be examples. It is acknowledged that the stated category would always be used *along with* the others. The examples do, however, make concrete the abstract; they show the practical application of the six-category approach in everyday nursing practice.

The following exercises allow for three phases of personal development:

(1) Ability to discriminate between the categories.

Prescriptive	1. Whilst delegating nursing duties
	2. Advising people prior to discharge
	3. Enabling students to develop new skills
Informative	1. During the admission of new patients
	2. Reporting to other disciplines
	3. At ward meetings
Confronting	1. When anti-social behaviour occurs
	2. When incorrect nursing procedures are used
	3. During multi-disciplinary meetings
Cathartic	1. Whilst counselling relatives
	2. Whilst caring for the dying
	3. Whilst caring for distressed, depressed or seriously ill people
Catalytic	1. During ward teaching sessions
	2. Whilst counselling the perplexed or undecided person
	3. Whilst preparing a nursing process assessment
Supportive	1. During all nursing situations
	2. During all teaching situations
	3. Throughout all human interactions

Fig. 4.9 *Examples of nursing situations in which skills in a particular category are used.*

(2) Ability to use each category skilfully.
(3) Application of the categories to the counselling situation and to the wider nursing context.

Exercises to aid discrimination between the six categories

Exercise 7

Aim of exercise: To enhance discrimination between the six categories of therapeutic intervention. **Group size:** Any number up to a maximum of 20. **Time required:** Approximately 40 minutes to 1 hour. **Materials and/or environment required:** Room in which group members can sit in a circle.

Process
1. The facilitator offers a brief theory input and discusses the Six Categories as per Figure 4.7.
2. Group members in turn state a category title and then offer an example intervention, e.g., 'Catalytic intervention: Can you tell me more about what happened?'
3. The group decide whether or not the example offered is a true example of an intervention in the stated category.
4. When all group members have offered a category title and an example, a discussion is developed about the use of the analysis.

Exercise 8

Aim of exercise: To enhance discrimination between the six categories of therapeutic intervention. **Group size:** Any number up to a maximum of 20. **Time required:** Approximately 40 minutes to 1 hour. **Materials and/or environment required:** Room in which group members can sit in a circle.

Process

1. Each group member in turn states in the first person something they may say in a counselling situation. They follow the expression by 'tagging' it with a category label, as per the six categories, e.g. 'it is not possible for you to see the doctor to-day'—informative category.
2. The group decides whether or not the 'tag' is an accurate one in each case.
3. When all group members have offered an expression and a 'tag', a discussion is developed about the use of the analysis.

Exercise 9

Aim of exercise: To enhance discrimination between the six categories of therapeutic intervention. **Group size:** Any number up to a maximum of twenty. **Time required:** Approximately 1 hour. **Materials and/or environment required:** A pack of twenty-four cards: four marked prescriptive, four marked informative and so on through the categories. The pack should be shuffled. A room is required in which group members can sit in a circle.

Process

1. The facilitator passes the pack of cards, face down, to the first group member.
2. The first group member picks the first downturned card from the top of the pack and shows it to the group.
3. The group member then offers an example of an intervention from that category.
4. The group decide whether or not the intervention offered is a true example of the category on the card.
5. When the group is satisfied the card is placed on the bottom of the pack and the pack passed to the group member to the right.
6. The cycle 2–5 is repeated.
7. When all group members have completed the round a discussion is developed about the use of the analysis.

Exercise 10

Aim of exercise: To identify individuals' and groups' strengths and deficiencies in the six categories. **Group size:** Any number up to a maximum of 20. **Time required:** Approximately 20 minutes. **Materials and/or environment required:** 1. A handout, laid out as shown in Fig. 4.10, is required for each

SIX-CATEGORY INTERVENTION ANALYSIS: SKILLS ASSESSMENT

Please place a tick beside the TWO categories that you feel you currently use MOST skilfully. Place a cross beside the TWO categories that you feel you currently use LEAST skilfully.

	√	×
1. Prescriptive		
2. Informative		
3. Confronting		
4. Cathartic		
5. Catalytic		
6. Supportive		

Fig. 4.10   *Six category intervention analysis skills assessment form.*

group member. 2. A room is required in which group members can sit in a circle. 3. A flipchart or chalkboard is required, laid out as shown in Fig. 4.11. A room is required with a circle of straight-backed chairs of the same height.

Process

1. The facilitator gives each member a handout laid out as shown in Figure 4.10.
2. Each group member ticks two categories that they feel they currently use MOST skilfully and place crosses against the two categories that they feel they currently use LEAST skilfully.

	√	×
1. Prescriptive		
2. Informative		
3. Confronting		
4. Cathartic		
5. Catalytic		
6. Supportive		

Fig. 4.11　*Six category assessment grid.*

3. When the handouts have been completed, the facilitator collates the results of the assessment on to the grid shown in Figure 4.11.
4. Out of the collated results can be decided a format for concentrating on the development of particular categories that are identified as areas of weakness.

Exercises to develop specific categories

Prescriptive category

Prescriptive interventions involve giving advice, being critical, making suggestions and generally attempting to direct the behaviour of the client. It is important that prescriptive interventions are made caringly and in the true interests of the client. They should not degenerate into 'putting people's lives right' types of interventions, neither should they patronise or oppress.

Exercise 11

Aim of exercise: To develop the use of prescriptive interventions. **Group size:** Any number from 6 to 18. **Time required:** Approximately 1 to 2 hours. **Materials and/or environment**

required: Large room or various small rooms, straight-backed chairs of equal height.

Process

1. The facilitator invites the group to sit in silence for two minutes and to recall an incident from their lives in which they were given advice.
2. The group is then directed to divide into pairs.
3. Each pair nominates one of them as 'A' and one as 'B'.
4. 'A' describes the incident to 'B' and 'B' listens impassively.
5. After four minutes, the facilitator asks 'A' to reflect upon the following questions:
   (a) How well was the advice given?
   (b) Was the advice appropriate?
   (c) How would *you* have delivered such advice?
6. 'A' then ponders on these questions aloud in the presence of 'B'.
7. After five minutes the facilitator asks the pairs to exchange roles.
8. 'B' then relates their incident to 'A' and ponders on the above questions.
9. When the complete cycle has been completed, the facilitator invites the group to reconvene.
10. The group identify the factors which contribute to legitimate use of prescriptive intervention.

Exercise 12

Aim of exercise: To identify valid prescriptive interventions. **Group size:** Any number from 6 to 18. **Time required:** Approximately one hour. **Materials and/or environment required:** A circle of chairs of the same height.

Process

1. The facilitator invites each group member to offer an example of a prescriptive intervention, stated supportively, caringly and therapeutically.

2. After each intervention, the group decides:
    (a) Was the intervention an example of a prescriptive inter-
        vention?
    (b) Was the manner in which the intervention was offered
        supportive, caring and therapeutic?
3. When all group members have offered an intervention, the
   facilitator invites a discussion on the therapeutic use of prescriptive interventions.

Notes
This type of exercise is easily modified for *any* of the six categories
and is useful in helping to 'cement' the concept of a particular
category in people's minds.

Informative category

Informative interventions involve instructing, informing and
generally imparting information to the client. In counselling, informative interventions should be restricted to factual information
and, as with prescriptive interventions, should not be concerned
with 'putting people's lives right'.

Exercise 13

Aim of exercise: To develop the use of informative interventions. **Group size:** Any number from 6 to 18. **Time required:**
Approximately 1 to 2 hours. **Materials and/or environment
required:** 1. Flipchart sheets. 2. Large felt-tipped pens. 3. A
large room or various small rooms; straight-backed chairs of equal
height.

Process
1. The facilitator divides the group into small sub-groups of 3–4
   people, as appropriate.
2. Each group member is asked silently to recall two people from
   their lives:
    (a) one who gave information badly;

  (b) one who gave information skilfully.

Examples may be drawn from parents, teachers, lecturers and so forth.

3. In the small groups, group members identify on a flipchart sheet two lists of items:
   (a) the specific behaviours and qualities of the people who gave information badly;
   (b) the specific behaviours and qualities of the people who gave information skilfully.
4. After fifteen minutes the group is invited to reconvene and share their findings.
5. The facilitator helps to draw up the necessary behaviours and qualities of skilfully offered information.

Confronting category

Confronting interventions involve being challenging or giving direct feedback to the client. A confronting intervention challenges the restricted attitudes, beliefs or behaviours of the client. Examples of issues on which people may be confronted are identified in Figure 4.12.

Confronting interventions should always be offered supportively. They should show concern for the client and should be offered clearly and calmly. Because the prospect of confronting others often causes anxiety, the temptation is often either to:

  (a) become aggressive and turn the confrontation into an attack;
    or
  (b) 'pussyfoot', or timidly approach the topic without being clear what the confrontation is really about.

Direct feedback on behaviour, use of language, attitudes, etc.

Direct feedback on the effects of the client's behaviour on self and others

Challenging illogicalities, inconsistencies

Challenging unaware 'unconscious' behaviour

Drawing attention to contractual issues or questions of rules

---

Fig. 4.12 *Examples of issues for confrontation.*

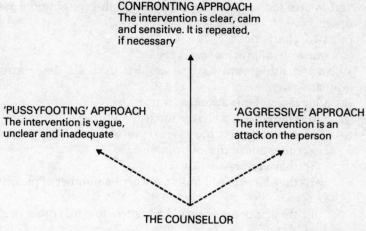

Fig. 4.13   *Range of possible interventions either side of confrontation.*

Figure 4.13 shows a possible range of interventions from aggressive through to pussyfooting and identifies confrontation as the centre point. Using confrontation, caringly, takes practice. The nature of the nursing profession is such that nurses often feel unable to assert themselves and confront 'cleanly'; as a result the outcome is often that they either attack or avoid. Courses in assertion training are frequently offered by colleges and extra-mural departments of universities and can be a useful means of developing confronting skills and further self-awareness.

Exercise 14

Aim of exercise: To practise the use of confronting interventions. **Group size:** Any number from 6 to 18. **Time required:** Approximately two hours. **Materials and/or environment required:** Large room or various small rooms; straight-backed chairs of equal height.

Process

1. The facilitator explains that this exercise involves role-play

and invites the group to break up into sub-groups and decide upon:

(a) two 'characters';

(b) one or two 'process observers'.

2. When the sub-groups have assembled the following instructions are given:

(a) One character is a student nurse.

(b) One character is a charge nurse.

(c) The student nurse has been reported to the charge nurse regarding one of the following issues:

(i) they are persistently late;

(ii) they have been abusive towards a number of patients;

OR

(iii) they have made sexual advances towards other members of staff.

(d) The charge nurse's task is to meet the student and to confront the student upon the issue. The charge nurse should be clear, calm and supportive and avoid either being aggressive or 'pussyfooting'.

(e) The process observer's task is to observe the role-play unfolding and rate the charge nurse on his or her ability to be skilfully confronting.

3. After the role-play has run for fifteen minutes, the facilitator invites each sub-group to evaluate their experience in the following manner:

(a) The charge nurse self-evaluates his or her own performance.

(b) The student nurse evaluates the charge nurse's performance.

(c) The process observers give the charge nurse feedback on the charge nurse's performance.

4. When the whole cycle has been completed, the facilitator reconvenes the larger group and invites feedback from the sub-group.

5. Following the feedback the group collectively identify what behaviours and qualities make for successful, supportive confrontation.

Notes

As this is a role-play it is vital that the people who have been role-playing are de-briefed after the exercise. This may be achieved by each 'actor' disassociating from the exercise by describing to the group one of the following:

(a) A recent pleasant experience.
(b) Interests away from the group and away from work.
(c) The house or flat where they live.

This exercise can be adapted to suit the particular nursing group taking part. More 'difficult' topics can be chosen for more senior groups.

The technical details of trade union representation and the grievance procedure do not normally go unquestioned in this role-play and can serve as useful material for discussion!

Cathartic category

Cathartic interventions involve enabling the client to relieve tension through laughter, crying, trembling or loud angry sounds. We tend to live in a non-cathartic society where the free expression of emotion is not often encouraged. In counselling and interpersonal encounters that take place in hospitals, it is important that nurses develop skill in helping others to express emotion.

It is asserted here that the free expression of feeling can enable the client to gain new insights into his condition, make him more productive, more spontaneous and more able to take charge of his life. Space does not permit a detailed analysis of the theory behind catharsis or emotional release and the reader is referred to Heron, 1977a for a more detailed and thorough account of the concept.

What may be said here, is that the process of emotional release tends to be self-limiting. If, for example, a person is 'allowed' to cry and no attempt is made to stop him or her prematurely, tears will naturally abate of their own accord. Too often, the person is comforted by a well-meaning counsellor or nurse who interrupts this natural process. The rule here then, is that emotions can be allowed to be expressed and need not be shut off too quickly. There seems to be a correlation between the amount of emotional expression that we can 'allow' in others and the amount of emotional expression that we can allow ourselves. If we can allow ourselves to shed tears, to express appropriate anger and so forth, we will probably be able to tolerate the expression of those feelings by others. Nurses who are frequently working with people who want and need to express emotion freely are often helped by first examining their own emotional make-up. It is here that self-awareness training is of clear practical value. Through becoming aware of and developing skills in expressing emotion, the nurse is able to support other people's emotional release.

There are a number of ways in which nurses can develop skills in exploring and expressing emotion in themselves and others. Co-counselling offers a simple and effective means of gaining cathartic competence; gestalt therapy workshops help in the process of handling personal feelings—both methods are frequently taught in short courses run by colleges and extra-mural departments of universities.

Examples of cathartic interventions are offered in Figure 4.14. All such interventions used deftly can enable the client to express emotion. All of them are also useful 'alternative' counselling techniques for helping to liberate new trains of thought, fresh solutions and different perspectives on distressing issues. Similar and other examples of cathartic techniques may be found in Perls, 1969a and Heron, 1975b.

Exercise 15

Aim of exercise: To explore emotional areas in group members' experience. **Group size:** Any number from 6 to 18. **Time required:** Approximately 1 to 1½ hours. **Materials and/or environment required:** Large room; straight-backed chairs of equal height.

Process
1. The facilitator explains that the aim of the group is to explore emotion and that expression of emotion during the exercise is quite acceptable.
2. The facilitator invites the group to divide into pairs.
3. Each pair nominates one of them as 'A' and one as 'B'.
4. 'A' talks to 'B', uninterrupted on one of the following points:
   (a) Early childhood experiences.

Type of cathartic intervention	Example
1. Giving permission	'It's all right with me if you laugh/cry', etc.
2. Helping to remove physical blocks	'Try taking three deep breaths; open your eyes really wide . . . uncross your arms and legs.'
3. Picking up on physical gestures	'Try exaggerating that arm movement . . . that facial expression.'
4. Noting mismatches between verbal and non-verbal behaviour	'You say you're upset and you're smiling.'
5. Repetition	'Try saying that again . . . and again . . .'
6. Contradiction	'Try saying the opposite of that.'
7. Catching the thought	Noting fleeting eye movements, facial expressions and inviting verbalisation: 'What's the thought . . . what are you thinking?'
8. Role-play	'What would you say to her if she was here now?' 'What would she say to you?'
9. Exploring fantasy	'If you could do whatever you wanted what would you do?' 'What would happen if you allowed yourself to do that?'
10. Mobilisation of body energy	'Stand up and stretch . . . shake yourself vigorously . . .'
11. Literal description	'Imagine that you are in that room now: describe the room to me . . .'
12. Reaching hidden agendas	'Who are you *really* saying that to?' 'What do you *really* want to say?'

Fig. 4.14 *Examples of cathartic interventions.*

(b) My relationship with my family.
(c) What I would tell you about myself if I knew you really well.
5. 'B' gives 'A' attention only and does not interrupt the content of their speech.
6. After ten minutes 'A' and 'B' exchange roles and work through the same process.

7. After all group members have completed the cycle, the group reconvenes and discusses the experience. There should, however, be *NO* disclosure of the CONTENT of the pairs' work. The discussion should centre upon the feelings of the group.

8. At the end of the allotted time, the facilitator invites each member of the group to describe something that they are looking forward to. This seems to 'lighten' the atmosphere and to end the session on a positive note.

Exercise 16

Aim of exercise: To practise the use of cathartic interventions. **Group size:** Any number from 6 to 18. **Time required:** Approximately $1\frac{1}{2}$ to 2 hours. **Materials and/or environment required:** Large room; straight-backed chairs of equal height.

Process

1. The facilitator outlines a variety of cathartic interventions as outlined in the figure above.

2. The group is invited to divide into pairs.

3. Each pair nominates one of them as 'A' and one as 'B'.

4. 'A' talks to 'B' and 'B' uses a limited number of cathartic interventions from the list. Only cathartic interventions are used.

5. Suitable topics are:
   (a) My feelings about my life so far.
   (b) My feelings about my family.
   (c) My relationships with my close friends.
   (d) My relationship with myself.

6. After ten minutes, the facilitator invites the pairs to exchange roles.

7. When all group members have completed the cycle of events, the facilitator reconvenes the group and invites a discussion on the experiences of group members. The CONTENT of what has been talked about is not disclosed. The focus of the discussion should be:
   (a) the feelings of group members;
   (b) the ease or difficulty of using cathartic interventions.

Catalytic category

Catalytic interventions involve drawing the person out through the use of open questions, reflection and empathy building. Examples of catalytic interventions are given in Figure 4.15.

Open questions	An open question is one that has potential for the client to develop. It does not require a 'yes' or 'no' answer. e.g. 'How do you feel about what's happening at home?', etc.
Reflection	Reflection is the technique of repeating the last few words of the client's utterance or paraphrasing what they have said, e.g. Client: 'I left home and found life became very difficult'. Counsellor: 'Life became difficult . . .' etc.
Empathy building	Empathy building involves the counsellor intuitively assessing the feelings of the client and verbalising that assessment. e.g. 'You sound very angry'; 'That must upset you a great deal', etc.

Fig. 4.15 *Examples of types of catalytic interventions.*

Exercise 17

Aim of exercise: To discriminate between open and closed questions. **Group size:** Any number from 6 to 18. **Time required:** Approximately 40 minutes to 1 hour. **Materials and/or environment required:** Handouts marked 'O.C.C.O.O.C.'; large room; straight-backed chairs of equal height.

Process
1. The facilitator discriminates between open and closed questions in front of the group.
2. The facilitator invites the group to divide into pairs.
3. Each group member is given a sheet marked 'O.C.C.O.O.C.'.
4. One member of each pair then asks questions of the other in

the order on the sheet (open, closed, closed, open, open, closed).

Suitable topics for this exercise include:
(a) The River Thames.
(b) The Sahara desert.
(c) Veteran cars.
(d) Steel tubes.

These topics are useful because they elicit short answers and thus keep the exercise brisk.

5. At the end of the first cycle of questions, the pairs exchange roles and the other person works through the list of question-order.
6. When all group members have both asked the series of questions and have been asked questions, the facilitator reconvenes the group and invites discussion on the process of asking questions.

Exercise 18

Aim of the exercise: To experience being asked a wide range of questions. **Group size:** Any number from 6 to 18. **Time required:** Approximately 40 minutes to 1 hour. **Materials and/or environment required:** Large room or various small rooms; straight-backed chairs of equal height.

Process
1. The facilitator invites the group to divide into pairs.
2. Each pair nominates one of them as 'A' and one as 'B'.
3. 'A' asks 'B' questions *on any topic at all*, continuously.
4. 'B' does not answer any of the questions but experiences the feelings that go with being asked them.
5. After five minutes, 'A' and 'B' exchange roles.
6. When all the group members have completed the cycle the group facilitator invites the group to reconvene and to discuss the experience.

Notes
This can be a powerful exercise for demonstrating how intrusive

some forms of questioning can be. The facilitator may want to invite the group to ask some 'risky' questions—reminding them that at no time are *answers* required!

Exercise 19

Aim of exercise: To develop the use of reflection. **Group size:** Any number from 6 to 18. **Time required:** Approximately 40 minutes to 1 hour. **Materials and/or environment required:** Large room; straight-backed chairs of equal height.

Process
1. The facilitator describes and demonstrates the techniques of reflection.
2. The facilitator invites the group to divide into pairs.
3. Each pair nominates one of them as 'A' and one as 'B'.
4. 'A' talks to 'B' and 'B' reflects appropriately. Reflection is the only intervention used. Any topic may be chosen.
5. After five minutes the facilitator invites the pairs to exchange roles.
6. When all group members have worked through the cycle, the facilitator invites the group to reconvene and encourages discussion of the difficulties and value of reflection.

Exercise 20

Aim of exercise: To develop a range of catalytic interventions. **Group size:** Any number from 6 to 18. **Time required:** Approximately 1 to 1½ hours. **Materials and/or environment required:** Large room; straight-backed chairs of equal height.

Process
1. The facilitator invites the group to divide into pairs.

2. Each pair nominates one of them as 'A' and one as 'B'.
3. 'A' talks to 'B' and 'B' responds with the following interventions ONLY:
   (a) open questions;
   (b) reflections;
   (c) empathy-building interventions.
   'B' attempts to use a variety of all three types of interventions. Any topic may be used.
4. After ten minutes, the facilitator invites the pairs to exchange roles.
5. When all group members have completed the cycle, the facilitator invites the group to reconvene and encourages discussion on their experiences.

Notes
A useful variation on this exercise is to invite the pairs to use the catalytic interventions as clumsily as possible! This should be followed by the exercise conducted as above.

Supportive category

Supportive interventions involve approving, confirming or validating the client's experience. The interventions should be genuine and appropriate and never patronising, paternal or maternal, neither should they be used 'automatically' as a type of positive reinforcement.

Exercise 21

Aim of exercise: To develop the use of supportive interventions. **Group size:** Any number from 6 to 18. **Time required:** Approximately 1 to 1½ hours. **Materials and/or environment required:** Large room and circle of straight-backed chairs of equal height.

Process
1. Each group member in turn receives validation from every other member of the group. In order to facilitate this the sentence:

'The qualities I like most about you are . . .'
may be used. The validation should be genuine and unquali-
fied.
2. When each member of the group has received validation from
every other member, the facilitator invites discussion on the experience.

Exercise 22

Aim of exercise: To explore self-validation. **Group size:** Any
number from 6 to 18. **Time required:** Approximately 1 hour.
Materials and/or environment required: Large room and
circles of straight-backed chairs of equal height.

Process
1. Each group member, in turn, identifies three or four of their
   own positive characteristics or qualities, to the group.
2. When all group members have self-validated, the group discusses the experience.

When individual categories of interventions have been developed, the group may take longer periods in the pairs format
attempting to use the whole range of categories. Alternatively
group exercises may be used such as the ones for discriminating
between the categories as described at the beginning of this section.

Once the exercises have been experienced, a commitment must
be made by each nurse to practise the use of the interventions in
the real situation; with patients in the ward or community. The
exercises are clearly of little value if the learning from them stays
within the group. It is vital that the interventions become incorporated into the individual's own self-presentation. Once this is
the case, the need to *notice* what interventions we are using
becomes unnecessary; the interventions have become the person.
Sometimes the transitional phase between first learning to discriminate between the six categories and successfully incorporating
them into self-presentation, is experienced as a period of clumsi-
ness and self-consciousness. Any new learning and any new skills
development must cause a change in the sense of self and such a

period passes into a natural, spontaneous sense of self which is broadened and deepened by the wider choice that is made available through the analysis.

What has been argued and developed in this chapter is clear. The skilled nurse/counsellor has self-awareness. They also have the specific skills of listening and attending. Thirdly they have skills in making suggestions, offering information, challenging, encouraging the release of tension, drawing out, and supporting. All of these skills need to be practised in an atmosphere of concern for and appreciation of the worth of the client. The development of these human skills through personal experience will enhance and enrich the nurse's approach to patient care.

These are the skills and qualities of the one-to-one interpersonal relationship. In the next chapter, the group process is examined and exercises in developing group skills are offered.

Recommended reading

Egan G. (1982). *The Skilled Helper: Models, Skills and Methods for Effective · Helping*. 2nd Edition. Monterey: Brooks/Cole.

Heron J. (1975). *Six Category Intervention Analysis*. Human Potential Research Project, University of Surrey, Guildford.

——(1977a). *Behaviour Analysis in Education and Training*. Human Potential Research Project, University of Surrey, Guildford.

——(1977b). *Catharsis in Human Development*. Human Potential Research Project, University of Surrey, Guildford.

Munroe E.A., Manthei R.J. and Small J.J. (1979). *Counselling: A Skills Approach*. Wellington, New Zealand: Methuen.

Nelson-Jones R. (1982). *The Theory and Practice of Counselling Psychology*. London: Holt, Reinhart & Winston.

Nurse G. (1975). *Counselling and the Nurse*. London: H. M. & M. Publishers.

Priestley P., McGuire J., Flegg D., Hemsley V. and Welham D. (1978). *Social Skills and Personal Problem Solving*. London: Tavistock Publications.

Rogers C.R. (1976). *On Becoming a Person*. London: Constable.

Schulman E.D. (1982). *Intervention in Human Services: A Guide to Skill and Knowledge*. 3rd Edition. St Louis, Toronto: The C.V. Mosby Co.

Tschudin V. (1982). *Counselling Skills for Nurses*. London: Bailliere, Tindall.

Venables E. (1971). *Counselling*. London: National Marriage Guidance Council.

CHAPTER FIVE

Experiential Exercises for Human Skills: 2. Group Skills

An overview of the group process

We all live and work in a variety of types of groups. If the counselling process as outlined and discussed in the previous chapter is comparable to any one-to-one encounter, similarly the group process is relevant to the study of any situation in which three or more people meet. In the nursing profession the individual joins many groups: the training group in the school of nursing, the nursing team on the ward, the variety of meetings, case conferences, and so forth. In these situations, the individual may play many parts and the group often causes that individual to act differently to the way they would in a one-to-one meeting. Various skills are required both to be a successful group member and to be a group leader. Before such skills are developed, it may be useful to have an overall map of the group process, as a means of understanding the stages through which every group, of every sort, seems to pass.

Figure 5.1 offers such a map, based on the work of Tuckman (1965). Tuckman noted that every group passes through four stages during its development and life. He described these as the stages of (a) forming; (b) storming; (c) norming; and (d) performing. During stage one, the forming stage, group members meet each other for the first time and attempt to discover what behaviour is and is not acceptable to the group. This is a time of 'testing the water', of discovering other people and, for the individual, of discovering their role in the group. In the 'storming' stage, group members characteristically become hostile to one another and there are battles between individual and group needs. In other words, each group member is trying to come to terms with how much they are to remain 'individual' and how much they are prepared to become at one with the group. Often this is a painful period in which there are fights for leadership of

Stage one: the forming stage
—the group meets
—members hesitantly get to know each other
—trust and disclosure are low
—there is minimal achievement by the group

↓

Stage two: the storming stage
—the group explores relationships between its members
—there is infighting and conflict between group members
—there are tensions between the needs of the individual and the needs of the group

↓

Stage three: the norming stage
—the group establishes 'rules' for itself: both explicit and implicit
—arguments and disagreements are settled
—the group becomes cohesive

↓

Stage four: the performing stage
—the group becomes mature and productive
—group members accept individual differences between them
—the group can work together
—the group has 'come of age'

Fig. 5.1   *An overview of the group life cycle* (after Tuckman, 1965).

the group or attempts at establishing a pecking order. Nurses in training may notice the advent of the 'storming' stage developing once an introductory block has become established or during the first year of their training. In this stage, friendships and loyalties are tested and it may be a period when certain individuals opt out of the group altogether and leave training.

Out of the storming stage develops the 'norming' stage, when the group comes to terms with itself and the individuals in it resolve their conflicts—both personal and interpersonal. In this stage, rules, both written and unwritten, are established and the group becomes more cohesive. Members typically get to know one another better and a more trusting, intimate atmosphere develops. Nurse training courses, when they reach this stage, are often perceived as having established themselves by their tutors and fellow nurses; the group themselves feel that they have arrived!

The norming stage leads on to the most productive phase of group life: the 'performing' stage. Here the group has developed a mature collective identity and its members are able to work easily and usefully together. In terms of nurse training, learners in this stage often sense a feeling of personal development through the group experience. One danger in this stage is that group members can be lulled into a sense of complacency through their satisfaction with group membership. This can be seen in certain ward teams where everyone has worked together for a considerable period and come to know and understand each other well. Such a group can become inward-looking and reject both new ideas and new members. Students arriving in such groups often feel left out or a sense of intruding. The group that arrives at the performing stage needs to keep itself alert to changes and suggestions from outside of itself. 'Groupthink', the term sometimes used to describe the tendency for groups to work as if they were closed-minded individuals, can occur if the group does not remain in touch and awake to other groups. It could be argued that many nursing groups and perhaps the profession itself, as a group, is on occasions guilty of such closed thinking.

This then is the typical cycle through which every group seems to pass. It may be viewed as a life-cycle of the group and is directly comparable to the life-cycle of the individual: it mimics childhood, adolescence, young adulthood and maturity. Thus the cycle of life as experienced by the individual is played out in the larger arena of the group. Viewed in this light, the group experiences can be valuable for developing further individual awareness. The person who monitors their behaviour and responses in the group can gain great insight into themselves through appreciating this correlation between the individual cycle and the group cycle. The nurse in the group will often see themselves 'reliving' stages of their own lives when they join that group. The group is perhaps the most potent medium through which to develop self-awareness. In the group both self-disclosure and feedback from others are present—two vital ingredients for awareness.

If the metaphor of the life-cycle of a group is accepted, it will be

understood that a group may well reach the point where it has ful-
filled its function and the group is disbanded. The cycle has been
completed. In nurse training this ending of the group life comes
naturally at the end of the three-year training period because the
life period of the group has been predetermined by the examining
bodies. In other groups, however, such a time period may not be
so clear cut and it is important that at periods throughout any
'performing' period, the group reviews its performance and function. Clearly, there is little value in continuing a group's existence
when the point of its existence has been exhausted.

Second to the issue of the group's stages comes the question of
the processes that occur during the group's life. Group processes
or 'dynamics' may be described simply, as what it is that groups or
group members do. Such processes occur in all groups of all types.
They are more noticeable in small, intimate groups, but also occur in professional and work groups. They have been so frequently noted that they are easily described. Figure 5.2 outlines a
variety of typical group processes that occur. Recognition of such
processes are vital for anyone running groups and are valuable for
the group member to become aware of. Once again, developing
such awareness is part of the larger task of developing personal
awareness.

Pairing as a group process can be noted when two individual
group members, usually sitting next to each other, engage in a
quiet and often hesitant conversation with each other. The conversation may occur as a series of 'asides' and can be a distraction
for other group members. It can occur as a result of disaffection
with the group, insecurity on the part of one or both of the pair
involved, or as a means of testing group leadership. Another form
of pairing can be seen when two group members form a fairly
exclusive relationship and support each other in a determined
manner whenever either of them makes a contribution to group
affairs.

Projection occurs when an individual identifies the group as
being responsible for their feelings. The person sees a quality in
the group which is, in fact, a quality of their own but of which
they are unaware. Thus the individual may say 'this group is hostile and unfriendly', when it is plain to the rest of the group that
such a description fits the group member themselves. Such projections may arise out of insecurity in the group or out of the individual's lack of awareness. The process of 'owning' projections, of

1. Pairing:	Two group members talk to each other rather than to the group.

2. Projection:	Group members blame 'the group' for the way they are feeling, rather than owning the feeling.

3. Scapegoating:	The group picks out one member to act as the person on whom to take out their hostile feelings.

4. Shutting down:	A group member cuts themselves off from the group and becomes isolated and often emotionally distraught.

5. Rescuing:	A group member constantly serves as the person who defends other members from attack.

6. Flight:	The group avoids serious issues by taking avoiding action: talking lightheartedly, intellectualising or changing the topic.

Fig. 5.2 *Examples of group processes or dynamics* (adapted from Heron, 1973b and Bion, 1961).

taking responsibility for oneself can be a particularly valuable piece of experiential learning in the group.

Scapegoating often occurs during the 'storming' stage of the group. The group looks for someone to blame for the way they are feeling and behaving and chooses a fairly quiet or vulnerable member on whom to vent their feelings. Alternatively, the group finds an outside scapegoat and blames 'the organisation' or 'the profession' for the circumstances in which it finds itself. Recognition of such scapegoating is part of the group leader's role and identification of it by the group itself can increase a sense of group cohesion and personal awareness.

When a group member becomes 'shut down' (Heron, 1973b), they cut themselves off from the rest of the group, often feeling swamped by it and emotionally fragile. Again, the skilled group leader notices such shutting down and helps the individual either to express their feelings or quietly to rejoin the group. Shutting down often occurs when a member begins to face important emotional issues that have previously been avoided. The shut-down person is in crisis: they cannot face their feelings and they cannot verbalise how they feel. Working through such a phase can lead to increased insight and the ability to handle such situations more successfully in the future.

The person who 'rescues' may be described as a 'compulsive helper'. They find it easier to defend others from attack than to let those people fend for themselves and to gain from the experience of doing so. Often rescuing others is a means of avoiding dealing with personal problems: to be seen as a person who always comes to another's aid can serve as a useful smokescreen for covering unresolved conflicts. Could it be that many nurses are compulsive carers and 'rescue' their patients as a means of avoiding looking too closely at their own affairs? Looking after others can mean that we ignore ourselves. Part of the process of developing self-awareness includes our standing back and enabling others to learn through experience rather than rushing in and helping too quickly. Often the temptation is to protect others from that which we cannot take ourselves. As we gain awareness and resilience, we can 'allow' others to live through their own lives without being over-protected or denied the chance to develop their own coping skills. This applies to a wide range of nursing situations: the patient who learns to cope with their anxiety develops the ability to cope with it again; the person who is allowed to live through a certain amount of pain, develops the ability to deal with pain. If we constantly 'rescue', we constantly deny people the ability to develop autonomy.

The group process known as flight can be demonstrated in various ways. The group which avoids difficult issues or decisions can be said to be taking flight. The individual group member who is constantly humorous and lighthearted may be taking flight in humour. The member who always has a theoretical explanation for everything is often escaping from feelings. Yet another form of flight is keeping group discussions and meetings on a superficial level, thus deeper and, perhaps, more disturbing issues are kept safely at a distance. Working through or avoiding flight are means of helping the group to grow. Self-disclosure occurs more readily when flight is avoided and group members are able to share each others' experiences and to learn from them.

Finally, in looking at the group process, it is worth noting that the energy level of any group will fluctuate from time to time just as the individual's energy level will have its peaks and troughs. Part of the development of group life involves living through periods of low energy and taking advantage of, and making constructive use of, periods of high energy. Again, the skilful leader and skilful group member will both *notice* such fluctuations, take responsibility for them and make adjustments as necessary.

Clearly, the theoretical and practical issues involved in group work are numerous. The recommended reading list at the end of this chapter includes books that take the above concepts further and deeper. It must be stressed that a theoretical understanding of the nature of groups is important for anyone who wishes to work with groups on a regular and serious basis. Practical experience of groups is also vital but this aspect is far easier to manage. As we have noted, we are all involved in group work throughout our professional lives; it is up to us to notice and be aware of the changing patterns and varying natures of those groups. It is through such observation that we learn how people live and interact together.

In order to highlight some of the aspects of group work, the following exercises explore (a) the group experience from the point of view of being a member, and (b) group facilitation. These exercises may be followed through systematically or specific ones chosen to highlight or experience a particular aspect of group work. It is often useful if these exercises are preceded by one or two 'icebreaker' exercises in order to help the group to relax and settle into the atmosphere of the session.

Exercises in group membership

In the following exercises, a clear aim is offered for each. This aim may be disclosed to the group before carrying out the exercise or, more usefully perhaps, the group is offered the exercise and decides upon its value after the event. Sometimes to disclose an aim is to pre-empt the group's own learning from the experience of a particular exercise. If, however, a group member or members specifically ask for the point of the exercise, the facilitator should offer the aim as one possible reason for doing it.

Exercises similar to and variants of the following exercises may be found in a variety of sources. See, for example, Canfield and Wells, 1976; Heron, 1973b; Lewis and Streitfield, 1971; Malamud and Machover, 1965; Stevens, 1971.

As was the case with the exercises in the previous chapter, it is important that participation in the group exercises is voluntary. If any member requests not to take part, such a request should be honoured. The member who chooses not to take part in this way may usefully serve as a process-observer and offer feedback to the group once an exercise has been completed.

Exercise 23

Aim of exercise: To explore the relationship and perceptions of group members. **Group size:** Any number between 6 and 12. **Time required:** Approximately 40 minutes. **Materials and/or environment required:** Circle of straight-backed chairs of the same height.

Process
1. The group facilitator explains the exercise as follows:
   Each group member arranges the rest of the group in order to form a family (e.g., 'David would be my father, Sue my sister, John my cousin', etc.)
2. When each group member has developed a family in this way, the facilitator develops a discussion of the exercise by asking:
   (a) what group members felt about their allocated 'family' roles;
   (b) to what degree the exercise highlighted particular roles played by group members.

Exercise 24

Aim of exercise: To develop group relationships and to highlight the occurrence of group dynamics and processes. **Group size:** Any number between 6 and 18. **Time required:** Approximately 1 to 1½ hours. **Materials and/or environment required:** Circle of straight-backed chairs of same height.

Process
1. The group facilitator invites the group to discuss one of the following topics:
   (a) The qualities of the caring nurse.
   (b) The qualities of friendship.
   (c) My relationship with myself.
2. The group is invited to observe the following rules:
   (a) Speak in the 'first person' (say 'I', rather than 'you', 'we' or 'people').
   (b) Speak directly to others (say 'I don't agree with you', rather than 'I don't agree with what John says').
   (c) Make statements rather than ask questions.
   (d) Avoid theorising and explaining other people's behaviour (e.g. avoid statements that begin 'I think that John *really* means . . .' or 'I think that Jane is avoiding the issue . . .'
3. The facilitator indicates to the group *every time* a rule is broken and invites the group member to rephrase their statement.
4. After one hour has elapsed the rules are dropped and the facilitator invites a discussion on the effects of using the rules.

Exercise 25

Aim of exercise: To encourage giving attention to the group and listening between members of the group. **Group size:** Any number between 6 and 12. **Time required:** Approximately 1 to 1½ hours. **Materials and/or environment required:** Circle of straight-backed chairs of the same height.

Process
1. The group facilitator invites the group to discuss one of the following topics:
   (a) The need for self-awareness in nurses.
   (b) The difficulties of becoming self-aware.
   (c) What stops me becoming self-aware.
   (d) Any other topic.
2. The group facilitator explains that after one member has spoken, any other member who wishes to speak must first *summarise* what the previous speaker has said. They may then make their own contribution.
3. This cycle of events is repeated each time a member makes a contribution—the next person must summarise before adding their own account.
4. After forty minutes the facilitator suggests dropping the format and invites free discussion on the exercise.

Notes
This exercise can also be used as a listening exercise in pairs. In this case, one person in the pair must always summarise what the other has said before making their own contribution.

Exercise 26

Aim of exercise: To explore group dynamics without non-verbal cues. **Group size:** Any number between 6 and 18. **Time required:** Approximately 40 minutes. **Materials and/or environment required:** Circle of straight-backed chairs of the same height.

Process
1. The facilitator invites the group to turn their chairs around so that the group members sit facing outwards, in a closed circle.
2. The facilitator initiates a discussion on the topic of 'verbal and non-verbal communication'.
3. After twenty minutes, the group is invited to turn their chairs round and to share their experiences.

Exercise 27

Aim of exercise: To experiment with the concept of shared leadership of the group. **Group size:** Any number from 6 to 12. **Time required:** Approximately 1 to 1½ hours. **Materials and/or environment required:** (1) A small cushion; (2) circle of straight-backed chairs of the same height.

Process
1. The group facilitator describes the process as follows:
   (a) Only the person holding the cushion may talk.
   (b) A person wishing to make a contribution must indicate that they want the cushion, but must not speak.
2. The facilitator places the cushion in the centre of the circle and invites the group to discuss one of the following topics, observing the rules of the exercise:
   (a) The nursing process.
   (b) The need for strong leadership.
   (c) The concept of a leaderless group.
   (d) Any other topic.
3. After one hour, the facilitator suggests dropping the rules and invites a fresh discussion on the exercise.

Notes
A valuable method of developing group and individual self-awareness is for the facilitator not to suggest a topic for discussion but to allow the discussion to evolve spontaneously.

Exercise 28

Aim of exercise: To explore the effects of silence on the group. **Group size:** Any number between 6 and 12. **Time required:** Approximately 40 minutes. **Materials and/or environment required:** A circle of straight-backed chairs of the same height.

Process

1. The group facilitator invites the group to remain completely silent for ten minutes.
2. The facilitator breaks the silence at the end of the ten-minute period and invites a discussion on the feelings and experiences of the group during the silent period.

Notes

The group facilitator may invite the group to close their eyes for the ten-minute period.

Exercise 29

Aim of exercise: To explore group feelings in a symbolic format. **Group size:** Any number from 6 to 18. **Time required:** Approximately 1 to 1½ hours. **Materials and/or environment required:** Large sheets of white paper; paints, pastels or coloured pencils for each group member; a large room in which group members can spread out.

Process

1. The group facilitator invites each group member to draw an abstract or figurative picture of the group in any style that the member chooses.
2. On completion of the picture, each member presents their picture to the group.
3. The facilitator invites a discussion on the significance of the pictures, and invites comments on similarities and differences between the various pictures.

Exercise 30

Aim of exercise: To explore self-disclosure and risk-taking amongst group members. **Group size:** Any number from 6 to 18.

Time required: Approximately 40 minutes to 1 hour. **Materials and/or environment required:** A circle of straight-backed chairs of the same height.

Process
1. The group facilitator invites each group member in turn to complete the following sentences—a 'round' of the group is completed before moving on to the next sentence:
   (a) 'I am feeling . . .'
   (b) 'What I am not saying at the moment is . . .'
   (c) 'I could shock the group if . . .'
   (d) 'What I like most about this group is . . .'
   (e) 'What I like least about this group is . . .'
   (f) 'The topic I find most difficult to discuss is . . .'
   (g) 'I would be happier with this group if . . .'
   (h) 'If I could be anywhere else at the moment, I would choose to be . . .'
   etc.
2. After all 'rounds' have been completed, the group facilitator invites a free discussion on the exercise.

Notes
The facilitator may invite the group to choose their own sentences for completion, thus personalising the exercise for the group.

Exercise 31

Aim of exercise: To explore similarities and dissimilarities between group members. **Group size:** Any number from 6 to 18. **Time required:** Approximately 40 minutes to 1 hour. **Materials and/or environment required:** A circle of straight-backed chairs of the same height.

Process
1. The facilitator invites group members, in turn, to say:
   (a) who they feel is *most* like them in the group;
   (b) who is *least* like them in the group.

2. The facilitator asks that group members do *not* give reasons for their choices at this stage.
3. When each member has had their turn, the facilitator invites a discussion on the perceptions of the group members.

Notes

It is important that the facilitator makes it clear that what is being asked is who is *most like* and *least like* the individual member and not whom the member most likes and least likes! This is a considerable change of emphasis.

Exercise 32

Aim of exercise: To share positive, formative experiences in a group setting. **Group size:** Any number from 6 to 18. **Time required:** Approximately 1 to 1½ hours. **Materials and/or environment required:** Circle of straight-backed chairs of the same height.

Process

1. The group facilitator invites the group to sit silently for two minutes and for each member to recall three positive, formative experiences from their childhood or up to the present time.
2. The group members then share those three experiences with the group.
3. The group facilitator invites a discussion on formative experiences.

Notes

A challenging exercise for groups that know each other well is for each member to also recall three *negative* formative experiences. If this format is used, it is recommended that the plan is as follows:

(a) the group members disclose and discuss *negative* experiences and then
(b) the group members disclose and discuss *positive* experiences.

In this format, the group closes on a positive note.

Exercise 33

Aim of exercise: To explore members' perceptions of their position in the group. **Group size:** Any number from 6 to 18. **Time required:** Approximately one hour. **Materials and/or environment required:** A circle of straight-backed chairs of the same height.

Process

1. The group facilitator invites each member in turn to report to the group how they imagine the group sees them (e.g. 'I imagine that the group sees me as a fairly optimistic person with a lot to say and who sometimes talks too much!').
2. After all members have had their turn, the group facilitator invites feedback to individual members from the group.

Exercise 34

Aim of exercise: To experience a sudden confrontation in the group. **Group size:** Any number from 6 to 18. **Time required:** Approximately half an hour. **Materials and/or environment required:** Circle of straight-backed chairs of the same height.

Process

1. The facilitator tells the group that in a few moments they are going to ask one member of the group to stand up and tell the group everything about themselves, in great detail.
2. The facilitator allows a few minutes to elapse and asks for comments on how people are feeling.
3. The facilitator then discloses that he is *not* going to choose someone to talk.
4. The facilitator then invites a discussion on the effects of the confrontation and subsequent withdrawal.

Exercise 35

Aim of exercise: To explore self-disclosure and group decision making. **Group size:** Any number from 6 to 18. **Time required:** Approximately 40 minutes to 1 hour. **Materials and/or environment required:** Sheets of lined paper for each group member. A circle of straight-backed chairs of the same height.

Process
1. The facilitator invites each group member to write down three topics that they would find very difficult to discuss. No further instructions are given.
2. When all members have finished writing the facilitator invites the group to decide democratically what is to be done with the sheets of paper.
3. When a decision has been reached, the group acts upon the decision. They may, for instance, choose to:
   (a) tear up the sheets;
   (b) read out the items on the sheets;
   (c) pile the sheets in the middle of the group and pick up someone else's sheet—the contents of that sheet can then be read aloud;
   (d) disclose one item from the sheet;
   (e) modify the sheets in some way.
4. After the process has been completed, the facilitator invites a discussion on the exercise.

Exercise 36

Aim of exercise: To experience being asked questions by other group members and self-disclosing to the group. **Group size:** Any number from 6 to 18. **Time required:** Approximately 1 to 1½ hours. **Materials and/or environment required:** A circle of straight-backed chairs of the same height.

Process
1. The facilitator explains that each group member, including him- or herself, will spend three minutes in the 'hot seat'. During this period they may be asked questions on any topic by other members of the group. The individual in the hot seat may choose to 'pass' on any question.
2. After the three minutes has passed, the individual names another group member to take the hot seat until all group members have taken part.
3. At the end of the process, the facilitator invites a discussion on the group's experience of the exercise.

Exercise 37

Aim of exercise: To explore the use of touch in a group setting. **Group size:** Any number from 6 to 18. **Time required:** Approximately 40 minutes to 1 hour. **Materials and/or environment required:** Blindfolds. Large carpeted room with large empty space in centre.

Process
1. The facilitator invites the group to put on blindfolds.
2. The facilitator invites the group to wander silently around the room.
3. As group members meet, they are invited to identify each other by touch alone. Once correct identifications have been made, those identified can acknowledge who they are.
4. After all group members have been so identified, the facilitator invites the group to remove blindfolds, to sit down and to share experience of the exercise.

Notes
The facilitator should remain unblindfolded in order to ensure that group members do not hurt themselves through collision with people or objects.

Exercise 38

Aim of exercise: To identify relative roles and relationships of members in the group. **Group size:** Any number from 6 to 18. **Time required:** Approximately 30 to 40 minutes. **Materials and/or environment required:** Large room with space for group members to stand in line.

Process

1. The facilitator invites the group to stand up and to stand along an imaginary line, in the position that they feel they occupy in the group.
2. The facilitator may offer suggestions about the end points of the line, e.g.,
   (a) quiet . . . talkative
   (b) submissive . . . dominant
   or, perhaps more usefully, may allow the group to decide on criteria.
3. When the line has been completed, the facilitator invites individual members to make changes to the order of the line, as they see fit.
4. When the process has been completed, the facilitator invites the group to sit down and to discuss the implications of the line-up.

Exercise 39

Aim of exercise: To explore individual group members' perceptions of themselves. **Group size:** Any number from 6 to 18. **Time required:** Approximately 40 minutes to 1 hour. **Equipment and/or environment required:** A circle of straight-backed chairs of the same height.

Process

1. The facilitator invites group members to think of a household object *or* a piece of music *or* a book.
2. Each group member in turn is invited to describe themselves as

though they were that object, in the 'first person' (e.g., armchair: 'I am soft, large and often get sat on . . .', etc.).

3. The facilitator invites discussion on the experience after all group members have completed the exercise.

Notes

As a variation on this exercise, the facilitator may *choose* an item for each group member, thus:

(a) 'Imagine you are a piece of music . . . what piece of music are you? . . . Describe yourself.'

(b) 'Imagine that you are a piece of furniture . . . what piece of furniture are you? . . . describe yourself.'

Other 'items' that may be suggested are: a country, a book, a town, a poem, an animal, a statue, a period in history, a famous person, a car, and so on.

Exercise 40

Aim of exercise: To explore spatial relationships between group members. **Group size:** Any number between 6 and 18. **Time required:** Approximately 40 minutes. **Materials and/or environment required:** A large, carpeted room.

Process

1. The facilitator invites the group to wander round the room and to take time to find the exact spot where they want to sit.

2. From these positions, the group members are invited to share their thoughts on the significance of their positions.

Exercise 41

Aim of exercise: To share positive feelings for individual members and to enhance group cohesiveness. **Group size:** Any number from 6 to 18. **Time required:** Approximately 1 to 1½ hours. **Materials and/or environment required:** A circle of straight-backed chairs of the same height.

Process

1. The facilitator invites each group member to listen to a 'round' of experiences of validation from each of the other group members. If required, the incomplete sentence: 'The things I like most about you are . . .' may be used.
2. The group member being 'validated' receives the round without comment.
3. When all group members have taken part, the facilitator invites a discussion on the exercise.

Notes

If the group members know each other very well, a challenging exercise can be to invite *negative* feedback in the same format as above. The facilitator should ask for such feedback to be given tactfully and supportively. This version must be used with care and only with the complete agreement of each member of the group.

Exercise 42

Aim of exercise: To experience self- and peer-assessment in a group. **Group size:** Any number from 6 to 12. **Time required:** Approximately 1 to 1½ hours. **Materials and/or environment required:** Circle of straight-backed chairs of the same height.

Process

1. The facilitator invites each group member to assess their personal weaknesses and strengths.
2. Following this disclosure, the group member invites feedback of perceived weaknesses and strengths from other group members.
3. When each member has both offered assessment and received feedback, the facilitator invites a free discussion on the process.

Notes

This process can also be used at the end of a learning session as a means of self- and peer-evaluation. It is important that assessment and feedback are always offered in the order: (a) weaknesses, and (b) strengths, so that the process ends on a positive note.

Exercises in group facilitation

The term 'facilitator' has been used throughout this section to describe the person who initiates group activity or who leads the group in some way. The nurse tutor running a group whose aim is developing self-awareness is acting as a facilitator, as is the student nurse who sets up a peer learning group which meets to share learning or ward experiences. The nurse who acts as a facilitator needs to make some considerations about how to fulfil that role prior to meeting the group. John Heron (1977c) has described six dimensions of what he calls 'facilitator style' that are worthy of consideration here. Those six dimensions are outlined in Figure 5.3. It is not suggested that a potential facilitator must use one particular aspect of a dimension rather than another, but rather that such decisions will arise out of the *type* of group that is to be facilitated.

The sorts of questions that may be asked in relation to the six dimensions before attempting to facilitate a group are as follows:

(1) Does this group need to be *led* or can it be free-flowing and open-ended? (the directive–non-directive dimension).

(2) Do I need to explain what is happening in the group or can the group 'explain itself'? (the interpretative–non-interpretative dimension).

(3) Do I need to point out rigidities and repetitions in group behaviour or should I let the group sort these issues out for itself? (the confronting–non-confronting dimension).

(4) Will I be able to handle the free expression of emotion in the group (including laughter, tears and anger) or will I need to divert it to lighter topics? (the cathartic–non-cathartic dimension).

(5) Should I use exercises, games and set procedures to bring structure to the group or should I let the group organise itself? (the structuring–unstructuring dimension).

1. DIRECTIVE The facilitator clearly directs the group	OR	NON-DIRECTIVE The facilitator encourages the group to make decisions for itself
2. INTERPRETATIVE The facilitator offers the group interpretations of its behaviour	OR	NON-INTERPRETATIVE The facilitator encourages the group to interpret its own behaviour
3. CONFRONTING The facilitator interrupts rigid repetitive forms of group behaviour	OR	NON-CONFRONTING The facilitator encourages the group to confront itself or each other
4. CATHARTIC The facilitator encourages the release of emotions in the group	OR	NON-CATHARTIC The facilitator steers the group into less emotional territory
5. STRUCTURING The facilitator uses games, exercises to bring structure to the group	OR	UNSTRUCTURING The facilitator works the group in a relatively unstructured way
6. DISCLOSING The facilitator shares their thoughts, feelings and experiences with the group	OR	NON-DISCLOSING The facilitator keeps their own thoughts, feelings and experiences to themselves and plays a neutral role

Fig. 5.3 *Dimensions of facilitator style* (after Heron, 1977c).

(6) Am I going to let the group know my own thoughts and feelings as they occur or will I play a more neutral role? (the disclosing–non-disclosing dimension).

The nurse, tutor or trainer who considers these issues is developing the sense of 'conscious use of self' alluded to earlier. If these issues are clarified, the facilitator will be in a better position to act knowingly rather than blindly or unawarely. Once again such a person will be acting *intentionally*. To go to a group prepared in this way is to have considered the needs of that group. Not all groups are the same and not all groups will require the same sort of facilitation.

Generally, a useful rule for working with self-awareness groups is to begin with a directive, structured and lightly confronting approach and gradually to help the group to take more and more responsibility for itself. As the group progresses, the facilitator is on the one hand increasingly non-directive, unstructuring and non-confronting and on the other, increasingly cathartic and disclosing. Whether or not to be interpretative of other people's behaviour is a moot point, but again, as a general rule in self-awareness groups, such interpretations are best left to the individual and the group. Figure 5.4 summarises these points about group facilitation.

The general points that may thus be made about the nurse, tutor or trainer who is facilitating a well-established group is that they should not over-direct the group but allow it to develop itself; do not heavily rely on structured exercises, but allow the group to develop its own structure; allow the free expression of emotion and be prepared to freely disclose their own thoughts and feelings as an equal member of the group. They do not rush to interpret other people's behaviour but encourage individuals to make sense of their experiences. These points are in line with the philosophy of experiential learning so far discussed, which emphasises experience, reflection and the transformation of knowledge or meaning.

The exercises that follow allow for a systematic investigation of the six dimensions of facilitator style. They may either be used progressively and in order or one or two may be selected to develop a particular aspect of facilitation. As with Heron's Six Category Intervention Analysis (out of which the dimensions were

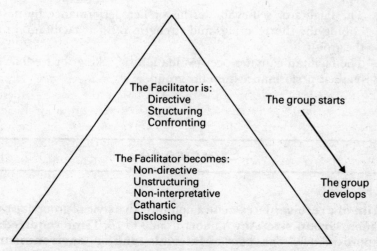

Fig. 5.4 *Appropriate styles of group facilitation for self-awareness groups.*

developed), the skilled facilitator is one who can freely choose and freely use any aspect of the six dimensions.

It is possible to combine the use of the styles of facilitation with the skills learned through the use of Six Category Intervention Analysis—Figure 5.5 illustrates the relationship between these two models. The styles of facilitation model outlines the general considerations that a group facilitator must make: the category analysis equips them with a range of specific *group interventions*.

Exercise 43

Aim of exercise: To exercise a directive style of group facilitation. **Group size:** Any number from 6 to 18. **Time required:** Approximately one hour. **Materials and/or environment required:** A circle of straight-backed chairs of the same height.

Process
1. The facilitator decides upon a subject for discussion by the group and keeps the group to the topic.
2. After half an hour the facilitator sums up and closes the discussion.
3. The facilitator self-evaluates his or her performance by describing the shortcomings and strengths of their facilitation to the group.
4. The facilitator invites peer evaluation by asking for feedback on their performance from the group.

Exercise 44

Aim of exercise: To exercise a non-directive style of group facilitation. **Group size:** Any number from 6 to 18. **Time required:** Approximately one hour. **Materials and/or environment required:** A circle of straight-backed chairs of the same height.

STAGE ONE: SETTING UP A GROUP

Question: What *general* considerations do I need to make about group facilitation before I start running a group?

Answer: Consult dimensions of facilitator style, and choose from the following dimensions:

Directive style_____	Non-directive style
Interpretative style_____	Non-interpretative style
Confronting style_____	Non-confronting style
Cathartic style _____	Non-cathartic style
Structuring style_____	Un-structuring style
Disclosing style_____	Non-disclosing style

Consider also:

1. Stages of group formation:
   —forming
   —storming
   —norming
   —performing

2. Group dynamics:
   —pairing
   —scapegoating
   —rescuing, etc.

3. Environmental considerations:
   —seating
   —lighting
   —ventilation, etc.

↓   ↓   ↓

STAGE TWO: FACILITATING A GROUP

Question: What *specific* interventions can I make when I facilitate a group?

Answer: Consult six category intervention analysis, and choose from the following interventions:

Prescriptive interventions	Cathartic interventions
Informative interventions	Catalytic interventions
Confronting interventions	Supportive interventions

Fig. 5.5 *The relationship between the dimensions of facilitator style and six category intervention analysis* (see Heron, 1975 and 1977a).

Process

1. The facilitator asks the group for a topic and allows a free-ranging discussion to develop, making no attempt to keep the group to the topic but allowing the discussion to evolve as the group wishes.
2. After half an hour the facilitator closes the discussion without summary.
3. The facilitator self-evaluates his or her own performance by describing the shortcomings and strengths of the performance to the group.
4. The facilitator invites peer evaluation by asking for feedback from the group.

Exercise 45

Aim of exercise: To exercise an interpretative style of group facilitation. **Group size:** Any number from 6 to 18. **Time required:** Approximately one hour. **Materials and/or environment required:** A circle of straight-backed chairs of the same height.

Process

1. The facilitator either decides upon a topic for discussion or negotiates a topic with the group.
2. During the discussion, the facilitator offers possible explanations for the behaviour, ideas or feelings of group members.
3. After half an hour the facilitator both sums up the *content* of the group discussion and sheds light on the *process* that occurred.
4. The facilitator self-evaluates his or her own performance by describing the shortcomings and strengths of the facilitation to the group.
5. The facilitator invites peer evaluation by asking for feedback from the group.

Exercise 46

Aim of exercise: To exercise a non-interpretative style of group facilitation. **Group size:** Any number from 6 to 18. **Time required:** Approximately 1 hour. **Materials and/or environment required:** A circle of straight-backed chairs of the same height.

Process

1. The facilitator either decides upon a topic for discussion or negotiates a topic with the group.
2. During the discussion, the facilitator invites possible explanations for the behaviour, ideas or feelings of the group, from the group members. The facilitator offers no interpretations of his or her own.
3. After half an hour the facilitator draws the discussion to a close, inviting a summing up of both content and process of the discussion from the group.
4. The facilitator self-evaluates his or her own performance by describing the shortcomings and strengths of the facilitation to the group.
5. The facilitator invites peer evaluation by asking for feedback from the group.

Exercise 47

Aim of exercise: To exercise a confronting style of group facilitation. **Group size:** Any number from 6 to 18. **Time required:** Approximately 1 hour. **Materials and/or environment required:** A circle of straight-backed chairs of the same height.

Process

1. The facilitator either decides upon a topic for discussion or negotiates a topic with the group.

2. During the discussion the facilitator draws attention to errors of logic, repetitive patterns of behaviour, interruptions and so forth.

3. After half an hour the facilitator draws the discussion to a close and sums up the content and process of the discussion as required.

4. The facilitator self-evaluates his or her own performance by describing the shortcomings and strengths of the facilitation to the group.

5. The facilitator invites peer evaluation by asking for feedback from the group.

Exercise 48

Aim of exercise: To exercise a non-confronting style of group facilitation. **Group size:** Any number from 6 to 18. **Time required:** Approximately 1 hour. **Materials and/or environment required:** A circle of straight-backed chairs of the same height.

Process

1. The facilitator either decides upon a topic for discussion or negotiates a topic with the group.

2. Before commencing the discussion, the facilitator invites the group to be awake to the occurrence of any errors of topic, repetitive behaviour, interruptions and so forth.

3. During the discussion, the facilitator makes no attempt to confront the group or individual members but allows the group to make its own confrontations.

4. The facilitator self-evaluates his or her own performance by describing the shortcomings and strengths of the facilitation to the group.

5. The facilitator invites peer evaluation by asking for feedback from the group.

Exercise 49

Aim of exercise: To exercise a cathartic style of group facilitation. **Group size:** Any number from 6 to 18. **Time required:** Approximately 1 hour. **Materials and/or environment required:** A circle of straight-backed chairs of the same height.

Process

1. The facilitator invites the group to embark on a discussion about personal or emotional issues. Clearly such a topic must be negotiated with the group.
2. The facilitator makes it clear at the outset that group members are free to express any feelings as they occur.
3. During the discussion, the facilitator uses cathartic interventions (see previous chapter) as appropriate.
4. After half an hour the facilitator draws the discussion to a close and to a lighter level as necessary.
5. The facilitator self-evaluates the facilitation by describing the shortcomings and strengths of the facilitation to the group.
6. The facilitator invites peer evaluation by asking for feedback from the group.

Exercise 50

Aim of exercise: To exercise a non-cathartic style of group facilitation. **Group size:** Any number from 6 to 18. **Time required:** Approximately 1 hour. **Materials and/or environment required:** A circle of straight-backed chairs of the same height.

Process

1. The facilitator either decides upon a topic for discussion or negotiates a topic with the group.
2. If emotional issues arise, the facilitator skilfully moves the topic on to a lighter note or invites contributions from other group members which moves the discussion on to a different topic.

3. After half an hour the facilitator draws the discussion to a close and summarises the content and process of the discussion as necessary.
4. The facilitator self-evaluates his or her own facilitation by describing the shortcomings and strengths of their facilitation to the group.
5. The facilitator invites peer evaluation by asking for feedback from the group.

Exercise 51

Aim of exercise: To exercise a structured style of group facilitation. **Group size:** Any number from 6 to 18. **Time required:** Approximately 1 to 1½ hours. **Materials and/or environment required:** A circle of straight-backed chairs of the same height.

Process
1. The facilitator introduces and explains a structured exercise to the group.
2. The group undertakes the exercise.
3. The facilitator invites the group to reconvene, as necessary, and to share their experiences.
4. After aspects 1, 2 and 3 above have been completed, the facilitator closes the session.
5. The facilitator self-evaluates his or her facilitation by describing the shortcomings and strengths of their facilitation to the group.
6. The facilitator invites peer evaluation by asking for feedback from the group.

Exercise 52

Aim of exercise: To exercise an unstructuring style of group facilitation. **Group size:** Any number from 6 to 18. **Time**

required: Approximately 1 hour. **Materials and/or environment required:** A circle of straight-backed chairs of the same height.

Process

1. The facilitator invites suggestions from the group as to any exercises, games, etc. that the group would like to undertake.
2. The facilitator may, as required, offer the role of facilitator to one of the group members.
3. The facilitator helps the group to undertake the exercise in the way they choose.
4. When the group has reconvened and shared experiences, the facilitator invites a summing-up from one of the group members.
5. The facilitator self-evaluates his or her performance by describing the shortcomings and strengths of the facilitation to the group.
6. The facilitator invites peer evaluation by asking for feedback from the group.

Exercise 53

Aim of exercise: To exercise a disclosing style of group facilitation. **Group size:** Any number from 6 to 18. **Time required:** Approximately 1 hour. **Materials and/or environment required:** A circle of straight-backed chairs of the same height.

Process

1. The facilitator shares a story, anecdote or personal experience with the group and develops a discussion around it.
2. During the discussion, the facilitator shares his or her immediate and/or past experiences with the group.
3. After half an hour the facilitator sums up the content and process of the group as required.
4. The facilitator self-evaluates his or her performance by describing the shortcomings and strengths of the facilitation to the group.

5. The facilitator invites peer evaluation by asking for feedback from the group.

Exercise 54

Aim of exercise: To exercise a non-disclosing style of group facilitation. **Group size:** Any number from 6 to 18. **Time required:** Approximately 1 hour. **Materials and/or environment required:** A circle of straight-backed chairs of the same height.

Process
1. The facilitator invites stories, anecdotes or experiences from the group and develops a discussion around them.
2. The facilitator encourages the sharing of experiences by members of the group but at no point discloses his or her own experiences.
3. After half an hour the facilitator draws the discussion to a close and sums up the content and process of the discussion as necessary.
4. The facilitator self-evaluates his or her performance by describing the shortcomings and strengths of their facilitation to the group.
5. The facilitator invites peer evaluation by asking for feedback from the group.

Through this series of exercises in group membership and group facilitation can be developed skills and learnings that may be carried over into any nursing situation. Combined with the interpersonal skills gained through the one-to-one exercises from the previous chapter, the skills learned may equip the nurse to be more awake, more sensitive and more self-aware. That self-awareness is the touchstone of all nursing intervention. The rest is up to the individual. Self-awareness is a continual, dynamic process that continues throughout both professional and personal life. It cannot be achieved simply through a series of exercises, but those exercises can spark off the process that, once begun, can carry the person forward to develop true human skills: the skills of compassion, caring and real interest in other people.

Recommended reading

Bion W.R. (1961). *Experiences in Groups*. London: Tavistock Publications.

Brandes D. and Phillips H. (1978). *The Gamesters Handbook*. London: Hutchinson.

Cartwright D. and Zander A. (eds) (1968). *Group Dynamics: Research and Theory*. 3rd Edition. London: Tavistock Publications.

Douglas T. (1976). *Groupwork Practice*. London: Tavistock Publications.

Heron J. (1977). *Dimensions of Facilitator Style*. Human Potential Research Project, University of Surrey, Guildford.

Johnson D.W. and Johnson F.P. (1975). *Joining Together: Group Theory and Group Skills*. New Jersey: Prentice Hall.

Malamud D.I. and Machover S. (1965). *Towards Self-Understanding: Group Techniques in Self-Confrontation*. Springfield, Illinois: Charles C. Thomas.

Sprott W.J.H. (1958). *Human Groups*. Harmondsworth: Pelican.

Schutz W.C. (1982). *Elements of Encounter*. New York: Irvington Pub. Inc.

CHAPTER SIX

Experiential Exercises for Human Skills: 3. Self-awareness Methods

The two preceding chapters have described exercises that develop self-awareness related to the counselling process and to group activities. This chapter explains some other methods that may be used to further self-awareness. They will enhance interpersonal contact in both one-to-one and group situations. They may be used alone or in a group. The experiential learning cycle should be adhered to as with the preceding exercises; that is to say, after a particular method has been used, some time should be allowed both for reflection on the experience and for future planning about how the learning gained can be applied to the practical nursing situation.

The methods described are related to meditation, relaxation, guided fantasy and body-awareness exercises. All of them can be repeated, and some are at first difficult. Repeating the exercise a number of times over a period of weeks and months can bring particular and lasting changes in self-awareness. No attempt is made to develop a particular theoretical framework around these exercises. The titles recommended at the end of this chapter offer a variety of theoretical viewpoints on many of the exercises contained here.

The serious student of meditation and of stress reduction is recommended to read these to develop their own understanding to a deeper level. The exercises alone, however, can serve as valuable means of becoming more relaxed. They also help to develop a heightened sense of awareness of the body and mind—including thoughts, feelings, sensations and intuitions.

Meditation

Meditation or methods of inducing altered states of consciousness have been used for centuries for mystical, religious and secular purposes. There are many excellent accounts of the history and theory behind various meditational practices (see, for example, Tart, 1969; Le Shan, 1974; and Hewitt, 1978). The following exercises are simple and effective. They can be used by the individual or by a small group. They are described as though they relate to the individual meditating on their own.

Exercise 55

Aim of exercise: To practice the meditation process of 'counting the breaths'. **Group size:** May be practised alone or with others. **Time required:** Periods from 2 minutes building up to 1 hour, once or twice daily. **Materials and/or environment required:** A quiet place where distractions of noise, interruptions and so on are within a tolerable level. The meditator may sit on the floor or in a straight-backed chair.

Process
1. Sit motionless, comfortably and with the eyes closed.
2. Breathe quietly and gently. Breathe in through the nostrils and out through the mouth.
3. Let your attention focus on your breathing.
4. Begin to count your breaths, from 1–10. One is the whole cycle of inhalation and exhalation. Two is the next complete cycle.
5. When the breaths have been counted from 1–10, begin counting the next 10 and the next and so on.
6. If you are distracted or lose count simply return to the beginning of the process and start again.

Exercise 56

Aim of exercise: To practice the meditation process of internal witnessing. **Group size:** May be practised alone or with others. **Time required:** Periods from 2 minutes building up to 1 hour,

once or twice daily. **Materials and/or environment required:**
A quiet place where distraction of noise, interruptions and so on
are within a tolerable level. The meditator may sit on the floor or
in a straight-backed chair.

Process
1. Sit motionless, comfortably, and with the eyes closed.
2. Breathe quietly and gently. Breathe in through the nostrils and
   out through the mouth.
3. Let your attention focus on the thoughts and feelings passing
   through your mind. Just notice them and let them go. Make no
   attempt to follow a particular train of thought or feeling: just
   notice and let go.
4. If you are distracted, gently allow yourself to return to the process of noticing thoughts and feelings and letting them go.

Exercise 57

Aim of exercise: To practice the meditation process of external
concentration. **Group size:** May be practised alone or with
others. **Time required:** Periods from 2 minutes building up to 1
hour, once or twice daily. **Materials and/or environment
required:** 1. An object of contemplation: a flower, a statuette, etc.
2. A quiet place where distractions of noise, interruptions and so
on are within a tolerable level. The meditator may sit on the floor
or in a straight-backed chair.

Process
1. Sit motionless, comfortably in front of the object of contemplation.
2. Breathe quietly and gently. Breathe in through the nostrils and
   out through the mouth.
3. Let your attention focus on the object of contemplation; concentrate on it and allow it to be the only focus of your attention.
4. If you are distracted, gently bring your attention back to the
   object of contemplation.

Relaxation

The following exercise encourages complete physical and mental relaxation. It may be used prior to the meditation exercises or on its own. Once the exercise has been learnt, it can be used in a variety of practical situations in the ward or the community. It may also be used to help anxious people to relax.

The use of a relaxation exercise may enhance self-awareness by drawing attention to the difference between our body when it is tense and our body when it is relaxed.

Exercise 58

Aim of exercise: To experience complete relaxation. **Group size:** Any number from 2 to 18. **Time required:** Approximately 40 minutes. **Materials and/or environment required:** A quiet, warm room in which participants can lie on the floor, undisturbed.

Process
1. The participants lie on the floor with plenty of space between each.
2. The following script is read by the facilitator at normal speed in a quiet but not 'hypnotic' voice.

'Lie on your back, with your hands by your sides . . . stretch your legs out and have your feet about a foot apart . . . Pay attention to your breathing . . . take two or three deep breaths . . . now let your breathing become gentle and relaxed . . . now allow your head to sink into the floor . . . your head is sinking and you feel more and more relaxed . . . allow your brow to become smooth and relaxed . . . allow your cheeks to relax . . . let your jaw relax and feel the tension easing in your temples . . . let yourself relax . . . more and more . . . let your neck and shoulders relax . . . now become aware of your right arm . . . let your right arm become heavy and relaxed . . . your upper right arm . . . lower arm . . . your right hand feels heavy and warm and relaxed . . . no tension . . . just relaxed . . . now become aware of your left arm . . . let your left arm become heavy and relaxed ... your upper left arm ... lower arm ... your left hand feels heavy and warm and relaxed ... you feel more and more relaxed ... your shoulders and chest feel relaxed ... your abdomen feels relaxed ... your pelvis and buttocks ... your right leg feels heavy and warm and relaxed ... your left leg feels heavy and warm and relaxed ... your feet feel warm, relaxed and very heavy ... your whole body is relaxed ... no tension ... just relaxed ... and you can appreciate what it feels like to be safe and warm and relaxed ... just lay back and enjoy the feeling of relaxation ... relaxed ... peaceful ... relaxed ... In your own time gently move your fingers and toes ... stretch your arms and legs ... now slowly sit up ... and appreciate the feeling of being relaxed.'

Guided fantasy

The following guided fantasy exercise incorporates aspects of meditation and relaxation. It may be used following either a meditation exercise or use of the relaxation script. It may also be used on its own. As with both meditation and relaxation, it can be used as a means of de-stressing the mind/body. It can also be a preliminary exercise in exploring the transpersonal domain (Tart, 1975; Heron, 1975a) or what have been called 'altered states of consciousness'. At a simpler level, it sometimes serves to put things into perspective, to help us appreciate our true position in the total nature of things. A similar, if more elaborate version of this exercise is described by Ram Dass (1977).

Exercise 59

Aim of exercise: To experience relaxation and to take 'time out' from the normal waking state. **Group size:** Any number from 2 to 18. **Time required:** Approximately 40 minutes. **Materials and/or environment required:** A quiet room in which participants can lie on the floor, undisturbed.

Process

1. The participants lie on the floor with plenty of space between them.
2. The following script is read by the facilitator at normal speed in a quiet but not 'hypnotic' voice:

'Lie on your back, with your hands by your sides ... stretch your legs out and have your feet about a foot apart ... Pay attention to your breathing ... now let your breathing become gentle and relaxed ... Now I want you to experience your body growing in size ... your head, your arms and legs ... your body ... are all growing ... experience your growing until your head reaches the top of the ceiling ... feel your vastness ... and experience a feeling of calmness and equanimity ... Now continue to grow ... your head goes up into the sky ... until all the surrounding town and countryside is contained within you ... you are continuing to grow ... You grow larger still ... feel your vastness ... until your head is amongst the planets and you are sitting in the middle of the galaxy ... the earth is lying deep inside you ... feel all this and experience the feeling of vastness ... of awe ... of calmness ... sit in this universe ... silent, huge, peaceful ... continue to grow ... until you contain all galaxies ... you are at one with everything ... experience the vastness ... the silence ... let everything be as it is ... Now very slowly allow yourself to return ... come down in size slowly ... past the galaxy ... down to the size of the earth ... now slowly to the surrounding countryside and towns and notice all that is around you ... Now continue to come down in size until you fill the room ... slowly ... gently ... Now return to your normal body size ... and just lie for a while and experience a sense of peace and relaxation ... think of your experience ... remain quiet and relaxed ... take a couple of deep breaths ... In your own time, slowly stretch, sit up gently and open your eyes.'

Body-awareness

The exercise in this final section is designed to increase awareness of body perception. It can be used as a means of relaxation and also as a method of becoming more acutely aware of body image, shape and size. Combined with the previous interpersonal and group exercises, it can round off the process of self-awareness development.

Exercise 60

Aim of exercise: To develop an increased awareness of body image and proprioceptive sense. **Group size:** Any number from 2 to 18. **Time required:** Approximately 40 minutes. **Materials and/or environment required:** A quiet room in which participants can lie on the floor undisturbed.

Process
1. The participants lie on the floor with plenty of space between them.
2. The following script is read by the facilitator at normal speed in a quiet but not 'hypnotic' voice:

'Lie on your back with your hands by your sides . . . stretch your legs out and have your feet about a foot apart . . . Pay attention to your breathing . . . take two or three deep breaths . . . now let your breathing become gentle and relaxed . . . Now I want you to become aware of your body . . . starting at your feet . . . Try to experience the feeling in your feet and toes . . . try to experience that as though you were *inside* your feet . . . Now become aware of the lower part of your legs . . . as if from the inside . . . Now your knees . . . become aware of the joints . . . become aware of your thighs and the top of your legs . . . experience them as if you were inside your legs . . . Now experience your pelvic region . . . now your abdomen . . . as if from the inside . . . Put your attention into your chest . . . experience the feeling inside your chest . . . Now your hands . . . your lower arms . . . your upper arms . . . imagine being inside your arm . . . Now experience your shoulders . . . feel the shoulder joints . . . Experience the feeling in your neck . . . the back of your head . . . Now your head itself . . . feel and experience your face . . . the muscles in your face . . . your lips, your nose . . . your eyes . . . finally . . . experience your scalp . . . imagine the feeling as though you were beneath your scalp . . . remain fully aware of all of your body . . . Notice which parts you can fully experience and which parts are numb to you . . . see if you can become more aware of those parts of your body . . . now just lie and relax for a few more moments . . . take a couple of deep breaths . . . and slowly, in your own time . . . sit up and open your eyes.

So the series of exercises is complete. The focus of the exercises has shifted from the pair to the group and back to the individual. In closing with exercises that centre on the self, I emphasise the theme that has been a recurrent one throughout the book: the development of self-awareness.

This book is only a beginning. It offers some methods of developing self-awareness. The hard work must be done by the reader. Out of the exercises described in the book, and in the references at the end of each chapter, will develop ideas for further exercises. Often the most effective exercises are the ones that you devise yourself.

It is to be hoped that the concept of self-awareness and experiential learning are clearer now and that the development of human skills can be seen to be possible. Such skills are at the very heart of nursing and form the basis for the development of a future, caring nursing service.

Recommended reading

Feldenkrais M. (1972). *Awareness Through Movement*. New York: Harper and Row.

Heron J. (1982). *Education of the Affect*. Human Potential Research Project, University of Surrey, Guildford.

Hewitt J. (1978). *Meditation*. Sevenoaks, Kent: Hodder & Stoughton.

Keleman S. (1975). *Your Body Speaks Its Mind*. California: Centre Press.

Kreiger D. (1979). *The Therapeutic Touch*. New Jersey: Prentice Hall.

Le Shan L. (1974). *How to Meditate*. Wellingborough: Turnstone Press.

Lowen A. and Lowen L. (1977). *The Way to Vibrant Health: A Manual of Bioenergetic Exercises*. New York: Harper & Row.

Naranjo C. and Ornstein R.E. (1971). *On the Psychology of Meditation*. London: Allen & Unwin.

Pearce J.C. (1982). *The Bond of Power: Meditation and Wholeness*. London: Routledge & Kegan Paul.

Tart C. (ed.) (1969). *Altered States of Consciousness*. New York: John Wiley.

——(ed.) (1975). *Transpersonal Psychologies*. London: Routledge & Kegan Paul.

REFERENCES

Alberti R.E. and Emmons M.L. (1982). *A Guide to Assertive Living: Your Perfect Right*. 4th Edition. San Luis, California: Impact Publishers.

Alexander F.M. (1969). *Resurrection of the Body*. New York: University Books.

Bailey C.R. (1983). Experiential Learning and the Curriculum. *Nursing Times*, July 20th: 45–6.

Bandler R. and Grinder J. (1975). *The Structure of Magic 1: A Book about Language and Therapy*. California: Science and Behavior Books.

Benson H. (1976). *The Relaxation Response*. London: Collins.

Berger G. and Berger P. (1972). *Group Training Techniques*. Aldershot: Gower Publishing.

Bion W.R. (1961). *Experiences in Groups*. London: Tavistock.

Bond M. and Kilty J. (1982). *Practical Methods of Dealing with Stress*. Human Potential Research Project, University of Surrey, Guildford.

Boud D. (ed.) (1981). *Developing Student Autonomy in Learning*. London: Kogan Page.

Brown R. (1965). *Social Psychology*. London: Collier Macmillan.

Burnard P. (1983). Through Experience and From Experience. *Nursing Mirror* **156**(9): 29–34.

——(1984a). Training to Be Aware. *Senior Nurse* **1**(23): 25–7.

——(1984b). Developing Self Awareness. *Nursing Mirror* **158**(21): 30–1.

Canfield J. and Wells H.C. (1976). *100 Ways to Enhance Self Concept in the Classroom*. New Jersey: Prentice Hall.

Cartwright D. and Zander A. (1968). *Group Dynamics: Research and Theory*. 3rd Edition. London: Tavistock.

Chapman A.J. and Gale A. (1982). *Psychology and People: a Tutorial Text*. London: The British Psychological Society and Macmillan Press.

Claus K.E. and Bailey J.T. (1980). *Living With Stress and Promoting Wellbeing: A Handbook for Nurses*. St Louis, Missouri: The C.V. Mosby Co.

Dewey J. (1938) (1971). *Experience and Education*. New York: Collier Macmillan.

——(1958). *Experience and Nature*. New York: Dover Publications.

——(1966). *Democracy and Education*. New York: The Free Press: Macmillan.

Douglas T. (1976). *Groupwork Practice*. London: Tavistock.

Egan G. (1982). *The Skilled Helper: Models, Skills and Methods for Effective Helping*. 2nd Edition. Monterey: Brooks/Cole.

Ernst S. and Goodison L. (1981). *In Our Own Hands: A Book of Self Help Therapy*. London: The Women's Press.

Feldenkrais M. (1972). *Awareness Through Movement*. New York: Harper & Row.

Francis D. and Woodcock M. (1982). *50 Activities for Self Development*. Aldershot: Gower Publishing Co. Ltd.

Francis D. and Young D. (1979). *Improving Work Groups: A Practical Manual for Team Building*. San Diego, California: University Associates.

Freire P. (1970). *Cultural Action for Freedom*. Harmondsworth: Penguin.

—— (1972). *Pedagogy of the Oppressed*. Harmondsworth: Penguin.

Heron J. (1970). *The Phenomenology of the Gaze*. Human Potential Research Project, University of Surrey, Guildford.

—— (1973a). *Re-evaluation Counselling: a Theoretical Review*. Human Potential Research Project, University of Surrey, Guildford.

—— (1973b). *Experiential Training Techniques*. Human Potential Research Project, University of Surrey, Guildford.

—— (1974a). Open Letter to Harvey Jackins. *Self and Society: European Journal of Humanistic Psychology*: No. 5.

—— (1974b). *Reciprocal Counselling Manual*. Human Potential Research Project, University of Surrey, Guildford.

—— (1975a). *Practical Methods in Transpersonal Psychology*. Human Potential Research Project, University of Surrey, Guildford.

—— (1975b). *Six Category Intervention Analysis*. Human Potential Research Project, University of Surrey, Guildford.

—— (1977a). *Catharsis in Human Development*. Human Potential Research Project, University of Surrey, Guildford.

—— (1977b). *Behaviour Analysis in Education and Training*. Guildford: University of Surrey.

—— (1977c). *Dimensions of Facilitator Style*. Human Potential Research Project, University of Surrey, Guildford.

—— (1978). *Co-counselling Teacher's Manual*. Human Potential Research Project, University of Surrey, Guildford.

—— (1981a). *Experiential Research: A New Paradigm*. Human Potential Research Project, University of Surrey, Guildford.

—— (1981b). *Assessment*. Human Potential Research Project, University of Surrey, Guildford.

—— (1982). *Education of the Affect*. Human Potential Research Project, University of Surrey, Guildford.

Hewitt J. (1978). *Meditation*. Sevenoaks, Kent: Hodder & Stoughton.

Husserl E. (1931). *Ideas: General Introduction to Pure Phenomenology*. Trans. Boyce, G. London: Allen & Unwin.

Jackins H. (1965). *The Human Side of Human Beings*. Seattle: Rational Island Publishers.

Jackins H. (1970). *Fundamentals of Co-counselling Manual.* Seattle: Rational Island Publishers.

——(1973). *The Human Situation.* Seattle: Rational Island Publishers.

——(1975). *Guidebook to Re-evaluation Counselling.* Seattle: Rational Island Publishers.

Johnson D.W. and Johnson F.P. (1975). *Joining Together: Group Theory and Group Skills.* New Jersey: Prentice Hall.

Jourard S.M. (1971). *Self Disclosure: An Experimental Analysis of the Transparent Self.* New York: Wiley Interscience.

Jung C. G. (1978). *Man and His Symbols.* London: Picador.

Kapleau P. (1967). *The Three Pillars of Zen.* Boston: Beacon Press.

Keeton M. and Associates (1976). *Experiential Learning.* San Francisco, California. Jossey Bass.

Keleman S. (1975). *Your Body Speaks Its Mind.* California: Centre Press.

Kilty J. (1982a). *Experiential Learning.* Human Potential Research Project, University of Surrey, Guildford.

——(1982b). *Self and Peer Assessment: A Collection of Papers.* Human Potential Research Project, University of Surrey, Guildford.

Kirschenbaum H. (1979). *On Becoming Carl Rogers.* New York: Dell.

Knowles M. (1978). *The Adult Learner: A Neglected Species.* 2nd Edition. Houston, Texas: Gulf.

Kolb D.A. (1984). *Experiential Learning: Experience as the Source of Learning and Development.* New Jersey: Prentice Hall.

Krieger D. (1979). *The Therapeutic Touch.* New Jersey: Prentice Hall.

Laing R.D. (1959). *The Divided Self.* Harmondsworth: Pelican.

Le Shan L. (1974). *How to Meditate.* Wellingborough: Turnstone Press.

Lewin K. (1952). *Field Theory and Social Change.* London: Tavistock.

Lewis H. and Streitfield H. (1971). *Growth Games.* New York: Bantam Books.

Lowen A. (1967). *The Betrayal of the Body.* New York: Macmillan.

Lowen A. and Lowen L. (1977). *The Way to Vibrant Health: A Manual of Bioenergetic Exercises.* New York: Harper & Row.

Malamud D.I. and Machover S. (1965). *Towards Self Understanding: Group Techniques in Self Confrontation.* Springfield, Illinois: Charles C. Thomas Pub.

Marson S.N. (1979). Nursing, a Helping Relationship? *Nursing Times,* March 29th: 541–44.

Maslow A. (1972). *Motivation and Personality.* 2nd Edition. London: Harper & Row.

Masters R.E.L. and Houston J. (1973). *Mind Games.* Wellingborough: Turnstone Press.

Moreno J.L. (1959). *Psychodrama,* Vol 2. Beacon, New York: Beacon House Press.

——(1969). *Psychodrama,* Vol 3. Beacon, New York: Beacon House Press.

——(1977). *Psychodrama*, Vol 1. 4th Edition. Beacon, New York: Beacon House Press.

Morris D. (1978). *Manwatching*. St Albans, Herts: Triad: Panther.

Munro E.A. Mantheir R.J. and Small J.J. (1979). *Counselling: A Skills Approach*. Wellington, New Zealand: Methuen.

Naranjo C. and Ornstein R.E. (1971). *On the Psychology of Meditation*. London: Allen & Unwin.

Ornstein R.E. (1975). *The Psychology of Consciousness*. Harmondsworth: Penguin.

Perls F. (1969a). *Ego, Hunger and Aggression*. New York: Random House.

——(1969b). *Gestalt Therapy Verbatim*. Lafayette, California: Real People Press.

——(1972). *In and Out of the Garbage Pail*. New York: Bantam Books.

——(1975). Group Versus Individual Therapy. In J.O. Stevens (ed.) *Gestalt Is*. Moab, Utah: Real People Press.

Pfeiffer J.W. and Jones J.E. (1974 and ongoing). *A Handbook of Structured Experiences for Human Relations Training:* Vols 1–ongoing. La Jolla, California: University Associates, Publishers and Consultants.

Pfeiffer J.W. and Goodstein L.D. (1982). *The 1982 Annual for Facilitators, Trainers and Consultants*. San Diego, California: University Associates.

Ram Dass (1974). *The Only Dance There Is*. New York: Anchor Press: Doubleday.

——(1977). *Grist for the Mill*. Santa Cruz: Unity Press.

Reich W. (1949)/(1976). *Character Analysis*. New York: Simon & Schuster.

Reyner J.H. (1984). *The Gurdjieff Inheritance*. Wellingborough: Turnstone Press.

Rogers C.R. (1967). *On Becoming a Person*. London: Constable.

——(1970). *On Encounter Groups*. Harmondsworth: Pelican.

——(1977). *On Personal Power*. New York: Delacorte Press.

——(1983). *Freedom to Learn for the Eighties*. Columbus, Ohio: Charles E. Merril.

Rolf I. (1973). *Structural Integration*. New York: Viking Press.

Rycroft C. (1972). *A Critical Dictionary of Psychoanalysis*. Harmondsworth: Penguin.

Sartre J.P. (1956). *Being and Nothingness*. New York: Philosophical Library.

Schulman E.D. (1982). *Intervention in Human Services: A Guide to Skills and Knowledge*. 3rd Edition. St Louis, Toronto: The C.V. Mosby Co.

Schutz W.C. (1967). *Joy*. New York: Grove Press.

——(1971). *Here Comes Everybody*. New York: Harper & Row.

——(1973)/(1982). *Elements of Encounter*. New York: Irvington.

Shaffer J.B.P. (1978). *Humanistic Psychology*. New York: Prentice Hall.

Searle J.R. (1983). *Intentionality: An Essay in Philosophy of the Mind.* Cambridge: Cambridge University Press.

Simon S.B. Howe L.W. and Kirschenbaum H. (1978). *Values Clarification.* Revised Edition. New York: A & W Visual Library.

Smith E.W.L. (ed.) (1976). *The Growing Edge of Gestalt Therapy.* Secaucus, New Jersey: The Citadel Press.

Smith P.B. (1980). *Group Process and Personal Change.* London: Harper & Row.

Stevens J.O. (1971). *Awareness: Exploring, Experimenting, Experiencing.* Moab, Utah: Real People Press.

Tart C. (ed.) (1969). *Altered States of Consciousness.* New York: John Wiley.

——(ed.) (1975). *Transpersonal Psychologies.* London: Routledge & Kegan Paul.

Tschudin V. (1982). *Counselling Skills for Nurses.* London: Bailliere Tindall.

Tuckman B.W. (1965). Development Sequence in Small Groups; *Psychological Bulletin* **63**(6): 384–99.

Whitehead A.N. (1932). *The Aims of Education.* London: E. Benn.

Wilkinson J. and Canter S. (1982). *Social Skills Training Manual: Assessment, Programme Design and Management of Training.* London: J. Wiley.

Woodcock M. and Francis D. (1983). *The Unblocked Manager: A Practical Guide to Self Development.* Aldershot: Gower.

Index of Exercises

Counselling Exercises

Index

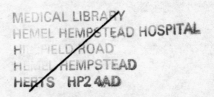